Choose Life

Where Personal Growth Meets the Stressful Reality of Modern Life

I0117627

Paul Johnson

chipmunkapublishing
the mental health publisher

Paul Johnson

Published by
Chipmunkapublishing
PO Box 6872
Brentwood
Essex CM13 1ZT
United Kingdom

http://www.chipmunkapublishing.com

Chipmunkapublishing gratefully acknowledge the support of Arts Council England.

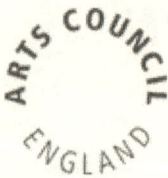

Choose Life

This book is dedicated to my wife Tara, without whom I would be utterly lost. You are truly the missing part of me. And to our astonishing and beautiful children, who have shown me just how much this life has to offer.

I would like to express my grateful appreciation to Geoff Thompson, for years of inspiration from afar, and more recently for his personal guidance, advice and encouragement. Without Geoff, this book would not exist. Thank you for helping me to believe in myself.

My thanks also to Neil & Keith Freeman and the boys at Goshinkwai Combat, my Mum and Dad, Paul Travis and the lads at Daisho Dojo, and the members of the forum at bohemiancafe.co.uk; all of whom have been incredibly supportive in so many different ways. Your positive influences have helped to shape both myself and this book.

The following people have been kind enough to allow me to make references to their work, and have all inspired and helped me on my journey so far. I highly recommend the following books:

- o Stress Buster by Geoff Thompson
- o Power vs. Force by David R. Hawkins (by kind permission of Veritas Publishing)
- o Action Meditation by Stephen K. Hayes - see website at www.mvmeditation.org
- o Heretic by Bernard Cornwell (and thanks for the words of encouragement, Bernard)
- o Easyway to Control Alcohol by Allen Carr (by kind permission of Arcturus Publishing)
- o Bufu Ikkan by Ben Jones – see website at www.japanesetranslations.co.uk

"The first step is simply that of self-honesty."

Paul Johnson

Choose Life

Contents

Spreading Wings

Learning to Fly

Choose Life

i.   Preface

The following pages chart the progress of an ordinary man's journey, a man facing the trials and tribulations of modern living, and finding real problems dealing with stress and anxiety along the way. We all accept stress as being part and parcel of modern day living - the high pace, the constant rush, frequently feeling run down and drained of energy. Often short of the ability to think, let alone cope. There is also the impact of stress on society around us, with growing dependencies on drink and drugs, increasing violence, road rage, stress related illness and disease, not to mention mental health issues. But what can we do?

First things first - this is not a 'how-to' book. It isn't packed full of techniques clinically proven to reduce your stress levels, and doesn't explain how to achieve personal enlightenment in ten easy steps or how to reach a higher state of consciousness in thirty days. What it does, however, is examine how much control we have, or even need. It considers how much of our frustration is due to the limited options and lack of quality that often appear to be our 'lot', and our growing awareness that there must be *more* to life, that this can't possibly be all that there is. If we are to get beyond this point, then our purpose in life has to be more than our base instincts of sleeping, eating and just getting through another week. Instead our expectations must go beyond the day-to-day drudgery. A sound philosophy to adopt for life is that *we must do all that is possible to survive, in order to experience everything that life has to offer.*

The journey charted across these pages shows how to find our own clear path through life, and uncovers one or two universal truths along the way. All of this is based on modern 21st Century living - a hectic family life with a focus predominantly on domestic issues rather than spiritual ones. It joins this domestic lifestyle with a few thoughts and principles from some of the Eastern philosophies, and finds that these two worlds are not separate and distinct from one another after all. That in modern times, real wisdom might indeed lie somewhere between the two. An unlikely direction? Perhaps, but this has come from the desperate need to discover how to cope now, in our busy and often stressful lives. Not halfway up a mountain in

Japan, sitting cross-legged and contemplating the universe, but right here and now, in what we laughingly refer to as the 'real world'…

So what exactly is it that we're aiming for here? Well, you know the moments of clarity that you get from time to time – it could be playing with your kids, or reading a book with one of them. It could be standing on a beach looking out to sea, or a moment shared with your partner, when the day to day crap falls away and you **really** connect. That moment where you feel both joy and peace, and say to yourself - *ah, this is what life is all about, it doesn't get any better than this.* But before long, the moment passes, the rush of day to day life catches up, and the pressures kick in once more. It doesn't get totally lost, but instead is forgotten, until the next time that we accidentally find the right frame of mind where we can see things as they really are.

I have found myself left with a vague feeling of loss, of some slight grief. Some sort of knowing that things should be better than this, but unable to find a context for this feeling, or know what to do about it. This has become my motivation - why can't we have more of this? Why should we only experience a few moments like this each year? Why can't we access this every day, and truly appreciate the wonders that are in front of us, that are in fact all around us? WHY?

We put huge efforts into juggling work, home, hobbies and interests, but generally accept that 'we are what we are'. If we were to sink even a fraction of our time and energy into discovering what really brings us happiness, then this could be a turning point for each of us, truly a life changing experience.

Having fallen apart, I was fortunate to stumble upon some simple but earth-shattering truths, which enabled me to rethink and rebuild my life. As I began to realise the significance of what I had found, that this was indeed a path towards real happiness and fulfilment, I felt a drive - an obligation almost - to share this experience with others. To share this in order to help friends and strangers alike to lift their lives without having to go through quite the same pain. If just a handful of people can be helped up from their knees by learning from some of my mistakes, then I will know this whole endeavour has been worthwhile.

Paul Johnson

Paul Johnson

Choose Life

ii.   Introduction

I've lost count of the pieces of good advice I've heard over the years: how to have a happy life, how to avoid being stressed, how to manage your time better, and so on - I'm sure you will have heard much of the same advice. Here are a few of the most common ones:

- **this is not a rehearsal, this is your life.**

- **no-one lies on their death bed wishing they had spent more time at work.**

- **the graveyards are full of people who thought they were indispensable.**

- **you need to take some time out for yourself.**

- **you just need to relax.**

- **you need to drink less.**

- **you need to drink more (!)**

I have to say that all of this was well meant, and much of it was quite sound advice. Especially the bit about drinking...

The trouble with good advice, however, is that no one seems able to explain how to put it into practice. Well intentioned (but often misguided) friends will fail to understand just how impractical their 'simple' advice might be when you're up against it. You might as well tell me to pull myself together, to just get on with it, I mean *where's your backbone young man???*

All the techniques, tools and coping strategies in the world are of little use if we can't make them work when it comes to crunch-time. There are endless techniques out there, and the temptation is to collect lots of different tactics and strategies from books, friends or wherever. However, when the brown stuff hits the fan, we don't know which of our dozens of techniques will best fit that particular situation. As a result, we usually miss the moment, and miss the opportunity to turn things around. Also, we generally have little idea of how our new-found techniques will hold up under the pressure of real life. I'm all for trying new ideas and strategies, but something here is failing us. Worse still, it's failing when we're already out of our depth, struggling to keep our heads above water and desperately looking for a lifeline.

Answers on a post card? Not quite. One of the problems with stress is that the truth is different for all of us. So, rather than looking for a perfect strategy in the usual 'one size fits all' approach, we need to find out how to help ourselves and discover what works best for each of us as individuals.

In writing this book, I claim no ownership whatsoever of the original ideas and concepts within. How could I? Wiser men than myself have known these truths (and many others) for centuries - an original idea is a rare thing indeed! Instead, this is a story of how the ideas and inspirations of others have been translated into real life. A life of picking an often painful path through the maze of stress and anxiety. A life of struggling through the realities of modern living, at times literally not knowing which way is up. A life lived alongside the feeling that somehow, somewhere, there should be more than this for each and every one of us.

My life.

Choose Life

WITHOUT A PADDLE

Paul Johnson

Choose Life

1.   Signed Off Work

It's difficult to pin point exactly when this all started, but it would be fair to say that things came to a head recently when I found myself in unknown territory - unable to cope with the simplest of things and signed off work with stress....

My feelings at the time? Blown away, devastated. Totally lost. In free fall, really, the first time anything like this has ever happened to me. Signed off with stress? *Me?* OK, so maybe I have been a bit strung out recently, and hey, I've probably been depressed at times in my life when some of the real shit has happened, but I got through that alright, didn't I? OK, so maybe I have been drinking too much, shouting at the kids and snapping at my wife, but even so, signed off work? I thought I was stronger than that. Much stronger. Do I really have to accept that perhaps the truth doesn't match up, that in fact I might be weaker than I ever realised? I'd always thought I was better than that - I mean, *anxiety*? Shaking inside without knowing why? Not coping with normal life? My god... what is going on here?

There was (and sometimes still is) a feeling of inadequacy that seems to goes hand in hand with this. We all work through some degree of stress - sure, that's ok. We all start showing cracks under the strain at times, not unusual. But *this*? We are into the realms of mental health issues here, and nobody, I repeat nobody, tells you that's ok. Come to think of it, nobody mentions it at all. It's definitely not coffee table conversation, and in fact is distinctly taboo for most of us. For me, I'm uncomfortable, ashamed even to admit that I might *have a problem* - I wouldn't dream of uttering those words out loud to the mirror, let alone to someone else. Oh, and I'm drinking a fair amount nowadays, most nights of the week if I'm honest. It used to lift things, if only for a few hours before bed, but now even this 'strategy' is failing to help. Worse, I'm feeling guilty about the drinking *and* it isn't helping. Not good.

Even so, signed off work? This is bad, I mean really bad. I remember seeing stuff like this happen to other people - being signed off with stress or anxiety. Sometimes even depression. I'm not an uncaring person, and each time a part of me would always be genuinely sympathetic to their situation. I would be thinking that these people are obviously going through a difficult patch, and no doubt there is an impact on those around them - family, friends, loved ones. And let's not forget that this is their health, their well-being that we're talking about here. Clearly this is more important than work. It's obvious that this is a big issue in the scheme of things, and if it takes a bit of time to sort things, then that's fine. Work can wait, we'll cover things at this end, so don't worry about it, don't give it a second thought.

We're all supportive around this - to be honest most of us are thinking *'there but for the grace of God, go I.'* We all understand where this fits in terms of priorities, work/life balance, all that sort of thing. So go on, get things sorted. Take the time that you need, and go do whatever it is that you have to do.

At the same time however, another part of me would be dismissing them as being weak, not able to hack it, not up to coping with a little bit of pressure. *Very poor show, eh?* Trouble is, I'm the one with the sick-note this time, and no doubt other people will have those same damning thoughts about me. What was it the Native Americans said, something about not judging a man until you'd walked a mile in his moccasins…?

Well, now it's me that feels uncomfortable about ringing the boss to explain. Now it's me that's worried about the idea of returning to work. I keep looking at the sick-note, wishing the doctor had written anything other than that dreadful word 'STRESS'. I keep thinking - what am I going to say when I go back to work? How I am going to explain? Actually… I don't want to go back, I don't want to explain. My god, how am I going to be judged? Besides, if I can't cope with the smallest of things at home, how on earth can I even think about managing the pressures of work?

But the sick-note does say 'STRESS'. I keep looking at it and checking. I must have gone back to it six or seven times by now, but it still hasn't changed. Now it's all official - I am incapable of coping. And I'm very uncomfortable with this. Worse still, as soon as I send the sick-note in, it will go on my record, and then there's nothing that I can do about it. A black mark on my record, an indelible judgement of weakness against my name. It's hard enough trying to handle what's going on right now, without also worrying about what it might mean for the future. Hang on a minute, what if I went for another job - I mean, that's one option, right? Find another job, maybe one with a bit less pressure. That would be positive, that would be a step forward, wouldn't it? Oh yeah, but then they ask for references. How many days off sick in the last 12 months. On how many occasions. And why.

Shit.

I'm not in a fit state to think about this. Things are bad enough right now as it is. My world is quite literally spinning around me. I'm at home in the kitchen, bent over with my head on the work surface (feels nice and cool). I can't think properly, and yet I can't stop thinking. It's all mixed up, doesn't make any sense - there aren't any patterns to it. A jumble of chaos and worry, all of it stacking up, more and more each minute. But I can't act. I can't do anything. Right now I can't even get my head off the work surface and stand up straight, let alone think my way through things. Especially not the future.

Can't stop thinking though. This is all going wrong, horribly wrong. Out of control... we're heading straight for the edge of the cliff here, so I've got to do something, and fast. There's only one thing for it - a tried and tested technique that has been used by generations of kids. One that's seen many of us through an impossible situation at some point in our lives. That's the one - fingers in ears, la la la, I can't hear you, la la la, I can't hear you, la la la.....

Straight up, this is exactly what I was doing inside my head. I had to act quickly to have any chance of stopping the downward spiral, and this was the only thing that came to mind. It seems comical now, but trust me, if there was ever a point where I have wondered if I was really and truly losing the plot, then this was it. No figure of speech here - I mean *really* losing my grip on this world, I could actually feel it slipping away, piece by shattered piece. One of the worst moments of my life.

Whilst all of this was going on, there was also a voice inside my head saying *"this is all wrong, you shouldn't be like this, look at you - bent over in the kitchen and can't move? It's pathetic. This is not how things are meant to be. You can't accept this as being ok, because it isn't. You shouldn't have to be like this, you have to take control, and get your life back before it's too late"*.

At the same time, I knew, *absolutely* knew, that this was beyond my capability. I knew that all I could do was try to get through minute by minute, maybe hour by hour. Forget about long term worries or consequences, forget about tomorrow come to that - it didn't exist. At that moment there was only 'now', and I had to get through by any means possible, however crazy, if I was going to survive.

La, la, la...

So I managed to get through the day. Not quite in one piece, but holding it together. Just about. Well, I was alive anyway, and decided to settle for that. The next morning I make the dreaded phone call into work, talk to the boss. Explain a little of what's happened (not too much of course, I've still got my dignity to hang onto), and do so in a fairly matter of fact way. I'm relieved to hear that she's more concerned about the state I'm in than anything else. Ha, and she doesn't know the half of it! Difficult to see how she could when I haven't told her the whole story... but anyhow, we have the conversation, she tells me to stay off as long as I need, and I have one less mountain to face.

So I stay at home. It's late July, and the start of the school holidays. I've been saying for months that I'll take lots of annual leave over the summer, so there's no problem with me being at home. If someone rings and I answer the phone, I'm just having some time off. Who's to know? This feels good at times, but I know that I'm just hiding. I choose not to think about this, to pretend that the thought hasn't even occurred to me, but deep down I know that it has. Deep down I also know that I have to face this. But not just yet.

Some of the time it's good to be at home - I've always worked full time, and ever since we had the kids there's been a pull to be around more. Well, I'm at home right now, the kids are full of laughter and the weather's beautiful. All the making of a gorgeous summer. I keep myself busy though, lots of DIY stuff that never got started, lots more that never got finished. It occupies my hands, my mind and my time. Gives me something to focus on - better to be busy after all, better than sitting and thinking. Feel things spiralling? No problem, lets drill, saw and hammer away. Kidding myself perhaps, but at least I'm managing to keep things at bay for a few hours.

At other times I slip back into the spiral. Terrible times. I'm lucky to have my wife around, as she will occupy the kids for a while, or take them out for an hour, give me some breathing space. Let me fall apart and then get my head back together without affecting them too much. This whole thing is especially difficult for her, as I've always been the logical one, the one that thinks with reason rather than emotion. The one that's always solid, her rock in the storm that she can depend on, no matter what. And now I've shattered into a million pieces, cartoon style. She is doing her absolute best here, but keeps looking at me, desperately trying to figure out what's going on. She can't understand how it is that her solid, reliable rock has fallen apart. It might be cartoon style, but it definitely ain't funny.

A week or two pass in this dreadful place of limbo, and I slowly begin to realise that the bouts of falling apart aren't getting any worse. In fact they seem to have levelled off. Not sure that it's improving, but I am beginning to get a handle on this, to see some sort of pattern, one that makes it bearable. I'm starting to understand what to expect in a day, and can now see that I have been through the worst and survived, that in fact each bout of spiralling does end. However uncomfortable it might be at the time, I can see a way through it, and that makes all the difference in the world. Ok, so this wouldn't exactly be my first choice of lifestyle, but despite not knowing how long things are going to be this way, it's becoming do-able for the first time. To be honest it's enough that the downward fall has stopped. It's better somehow to be rock bottom than to be in freefall - at least I know where I am, and that it can't get any worse. I find some twisted comfort in this.

Deep down I know that I've got myself wrapped up in some sort of cocoon, some sort of false version of reality, but I also know this is necessary if I am to survive. Not sure how I know this, but I do. I honestly can't see my situation getting much better, not in the near future anyway.

The trouble is that it's not just my wife who has been used to relying on my strength - I have too. For years I've known that whatever happens, no matter how bad things might get (and they have at times), I will not stop, I will not accept defeat, and I will never, ever give in. Only now I have. Now I've collapsed, and it's hard to see how I will ever be strong again after falling so very far. To imagine ever being solid again, being back at work, fit and well, able to deal with it all. Something has changed forever, and not for the better. I feel a sense of loss, a sort of grieving, perhaps, for a part of me that seems to have died.

Fortunately, however, fate decided to play a hand. This is one of those unlikely events that just happened to work out at the right time. To set the scene: some time ago I had been encouraged by a friend to write an article for his website. I decided to give it a bash, and to my surprise found that I had something to say. This quickly developed into an article which tied some basic oriental philosophy into the realities of modern living. I emailed this to my friend, and thought no more about it.

Somehow the article got overlooked, and instead of being put up on his website for the world to see, it sat unused, a forgotten file on a computer. A year or so later, I remembered, printed it out and reread it. Getting the feeling that maybe it wasn't a bad piece of work, I rewrote it, sharpened it up a bit, and started to think that it might be good enough to be published somewhere, to go on display for other people to read. Something in my heart told me that it was good enough, that it would make the grade. Something hinted at this being the beginnings of something greater, at perhaps even finding my true vocation. My fears and anxieties were quick to interrupt and drown this voice out, ridiculing me for having the nerve to have such flights of fancy. But deep down, the quiet voice persisted.

Two days before I crashed and burned, I was at work, full of confidence on an exhausted high. I could see the potential that seemed to be hovering in front of me, and for a few minutes I dared to believe in myself. Quickly, before doubt could take a hold, I

Choose Life

emailed my article off to a guy whose writing I had been following for some years. I sent it from my work email with a note saying - *'bit of a cheek, I know, but would you mind taking a look at this and see what you think?'* I wasn't entirely sure that I would get a reply, but sent it off anyway. Naturally enough I forgot all about this when my life came crashing down around me a couple of days later. It was hardly significant in the scheme of things. Or so you would have thought…

Fast forwarding to the end of my second week on the sick, I suddenly remembered about the article. I had a feeling something might have happened, that I might have had a reply from this guy. Can't access my email because I'm not at work, and don't know what to do. I go backwards and forwards with this, forwards and backwards, and eventually decide not to be so stupid - after all, who am I kidding? Mind made up, I ignore the feeling. But it keeps coming, so we play the game. I keep ignoring, it keeps persisting. Finally I give in, ring a mate at work and ask him to check my emails. He rings back a few minutes later to say yes, there is a reply from this guy. Time stands still…

I'm standing outside on the driveway because I've hardly got a signal on my mobile, and he reads it to me. The email says that my article is quite good, well written even. Wow! Hold on a minute, it goes on to say that if I don't mind, he would quite like it to go onto the articles page of his website. If I don't mind? If I don't bloody well mind?! Are you taking the mickey here, of course I don't mind! Woo-hoo!!

For me this was a fantastic moment. I'm smiling now as I sit here writing these words, remembering just how good it felt. This would have been great at any point, but to get such a result when I was rock bottom with absolutely no idea how I was going to get back up - to get it then was just out of this world. One of those things that just 'happened' at the right time, that you couldn't have dreamt up. This gave me a boost when I needed it most, and believe me, I needed it. I was still weak and exhausted, still wobbly from one moment to the next, but this was so positive and uplifting. An injection of inspiration and energy that I needed like a man in the desert needs a drink of water. Absolutely lifesaving.

I have to say though, that as fantastic as this was, it hardly got me back on my feet again. There was no quick or easy fix - I was too far gone for that. Mentally, I had been flat on my back for two weeks, following a build up of months, if not years. Receiving this good news did give me a massive lift, but it would be much more accurate to say that it got me back up to my knees rather than raising me to the skies. From there however, all things would become possible.

It turned out later that this same guy would provide more help and inspiration further along the path, although neither of us could have known this at the time. Still, this first gift was by far the most important, the thing that helped me to find my way again through the fog of stress and depression. And for that I am eternally grateful.

2.   The Hardest Fight Of All

It is all too easy to take out our frustrations on those we are closest to - we always hurt the ones we love, as countless songs have said over the years. Those who aren't able to defend themselves will often bear the brunt of this, as my own reflections have shamefully brought me to realise. I usually arrive home from work feeling a little frazzled from the day, but ready to see my family - catch up with them, get some time with the kids before all too soon they're off to bed. If I'm late home, it can seem like I barely see them before the next day comes around, the mad rush of the morning and then off to work again. It sometimes feels like being a part-time parent (with plenty of guilt attached) so I generally look forward to coming home, ready for us all to enjoy some time together.

Of course what tends to happen is that my tolerance levels are pretty low after a hectic day at work. After five or ten minutes at home, the noise is starting to get the better of me and my 'honourable' intentions have vanished without trace. Snappity, snap. Raised voices, cutting them off in their tracks. The nice family scene is quickly replaced by an air of thick tension and uneasiness. Not good, especially given the fact that all three kids and my wife were actually pleased to see me when I walked through the door. It takes a special kind of stupid to destroy this so quickly and effortlessly.

Of course, at the time you can't see that any of this is your own fault. It's always someone else, isn't it? Often it's the kids and their noise, maybe the dog is whining to go out, the lights are too bright or the TV is too loud. Anything. It's also easy to project blame onto your partner. Way, way too easy. Chances are they don't deserve any of this, but you can't see it. This is true enough if you're carrying a little stress, but when it's getting out of hand and those feelings have turned into a real millstone around your neck, then it takes on a different meaning. You continue to project blame and responsibility anywhere other than at your own feet, but now it's in the heavyweight league. Your 'truth' may be warped beyond recognition, but to you it's all clear and straightforward, and you can't see why others don't follow your logic - *for gods sake why is it so difficult for them to understand?!*

Of course, in reality it is difficult, because they are also busy coping with their own pressures, and as your own stress levels have built up, you have somehow dropped the close communication that you used to take for granted. Or to put it another way, the chances are that you haven't told them. Let's be honest here, it's not rocket science, is it? If you don't talk to your other half, how on earth can they understand or help? I know this sounds a bit like 'stating the bleeding obvious' (I do have a diploma in this), but when you're in such a state, believe me, you cannot see what is going on in front of your nose. You soldier on, doing your best, but despite these 'best' endeavours, still manage to cause upset and chaos on a daily basis. And worst of all, you fail to see the terrible impact you are having on those around you.

This really is the crux of the matter. However unlikely it might seem, and however un-dramatic it might appear - *this* is the turning point that you're desperate for, *this* is where the healing starts. All you have to do is be honest about how you're affecting those closest to you. Sounds easy? Sure, well it always does when you're just reading a line in a book. But this needs to be something more - so let's stop for a moment. Put the book down right now, and take just one minute out of your life to think this through. Be honest with yourself. No-one else can hear your thoughts, it's not like anyone is asking you to make an announcement on TV, is it? Ask yourself now - exactly what impact are you *really* having on those around you, by the way you're behaving or the way you're talking? Not to mention the destructive way that you're often thinking. How is this impacting on those around you?

There is something inside us all, which invariably tries to tell us that everything is ok. That it isn't all that bad. *No-one's perfect you know, all-in-all it's kind of ok, you're doing the best you can under the circumstances, after all you're only human...* Recognise that part of you? Well, sometimes this instinct for self preservation is invaluable, but right now you are going to have to park it, put it to one side, because it will only try to protect you from the truth and in doing so will stop you from being totally honest with yourself. If you don't have self-honesty at this point, then you have nothing at all, and any supposed progress or future development will be built on very unstable foundations. Without self-honesty your journey will end right here. Understanding this is absolutely vital.

You need to know the whole truth, and understand the full impact you are making on those that are close to you, irrespective of context, reasons or excuses. You *must* have this understanding if you are ever going to move on and grow. So, at the end of this paragraph, put the book down and find somewhere you won't be disturbed. It doesn't matter where, could be in the car, the toilet or wherever, but take a quiet minute, turn your mobile phone off and think it through. Just stop and weigh this up for yourself - **what impact are you really having?**

I'll say it again. All you have to do is be honest about how you're affecting those who are closest to you. You don't have to tell anyone (although it will often help), but you *must* be straight with yourself. Think about it - we all say that we would die for our children, and most of us would, but we can't control our temper when we're tired and stressed from work? Really? Is this harder than giving up your life? Well, in a sense perhaps it is more difficult, because this isn't some flash of heroic action, this is a long hard fight against an invisible enemy that we usually don't understand. This wears you down, and hits hardest when you are low and vulnerable. It takes real strength to fight this, and even though it may seem trivial, domestic or unimportant, isn't sexy and certainly doesn't win any accolades down the pub or in the dojo (training hall), despite all of that - *this is actually the most important fight of your life*. Never mind work - chasing overtime or promotions, building a career or bringing in a few extra quid. Never mind the risk of losing face amongst friends or enemies, never mind your reputation or social standing. Sure, it all seems important at the time, but when you take a step back and get things in perspective, you can see that there is nothing more important in this world than those you love.

You ask any elderly person what is important in life, and they all say the same things - friends and family. Not money, not work, not travel. Friends and family, people and relationships. These are the things that are important, so why wait until you are old and frail before you learn this lesson? Why leave it until you can only look back with regret?

Occasionally we do have moments of clarity where we can see things for what they are, but this is oh-so easily lost. We lose sight of these truths because they are domestic and day-to-day ordinary. In turn we are fooled into thinking they must be a fairly low priority, and that other more pressing matters require our energy and attention. This is what makes it so difficult, because we need to understand just how important this is, and not be distracted by false promises and mistaken priorities that would sidetrack us from life's happiness. This is what makes it the hardest fight of all.

In one of life's rather unfunny ironies, the battle seems to start in earnest when you are at your lowest, when you feel there is no fight left in you and you're ready to quit. Recognise anything of your own situation in those words? If so, then please don't give up, because you are not alone in this. Exhaustion? Anxiety? Despair? Doubting everything you ever thought you knew about yourself? Guess what - this is normal. Ok, perhaps not something that you share with every single person in the country, but this is much more common than you would ever dare to believe. Mental health problems? Slippery slope to the funny farm? Sure, if you want this to be your truth. No problem, one self-fulfilling prophesy coming right up!

You know the old saying – 'if you think you can, then you're right. If you think you can't, then you're right'? This motto is part of the home-grown philosophy that belonged to my grandparent's era. There are lots of similar such sayings and old wives tales - I'm sure you've heard as many as I have. Well, the older I'm getting, the more truth I can see in a lot of these sayings. I don't think this is just about getting older (I hope not anyway), there is more to it than that. This was a generation that was pretty tough, having lived through some real hardships including two world wars and years of food rationing. Out of this seems to have come an ability to cut through the crap and get to the heart of an issue. Not always very sensitively, granted, but that perhaps came with the territory. After all, this was a generation accustomed to concentrating on survival, on getting through, keeping going. Not like us softies today. I think many of this older generation are right in thinking that we often 'don't know we're born', and don't realise how lucky we are. Here I am, at the back end of my thirties, only just waking up to this realisation…

In the context of the slippery slope to the funny farm, with fears about mental health and self-fulfilling prophesies abounding, then that piece of advice - *if you think you can, then you're right. If you think you can't, then you're right* - really does hit the mark. If you think that you are going to keep falling - the initial onset of depression sinking inevitably into the depths of despair, or if you think you will end up ruining your relationships, or perhaps fear that you will never get back to work again - if you do believe these things, then there is a much greater likelihood of them becoming true. It seems that our Grannies might well have a point, but what their old-fashioned advice hasn't told us, is how to actually put this into practice. So what do you do? Where do you go when you want to get up off your knees but can't? When you recognise the truth in these words but lack the strength to get up and sort yourself out? What do you do then?

There is only one thing you can do at this stage, other than lying back and sinking even further. One course of action that remains positive, and is still realistically within your power to carry out. Yet it is one that many of us are uncomfortable with, and prefer not to do, even when we are teetering on the very edge, and know that we can't carry this weight any further on our own. But what exactly is this life saver?

ASK FOR HELP.

Sounds easy doesn't it? Well, perhaps for some people it is, but for me it's a real killer. I was brought up to stand on my own two feet, to be independent. Nothing wrong with that - it's been a very positive thing in general, and has undoubtedly been to my advantage for the most part. But like many things, it can be a double-edged sword. One side effect is that it can be very difficult to ask for help - even in simple situations where it really shouldn't matter. Worse, if help is offered, even by people that I know and trust, I will almost always say, *no, I can manage, thanks,* and press on alone, often cursing myself for not being able to accept that little bit of assistance. Something unhealthy in there for sure, feeling that you should always be able to manage everything without any help at all. Not good, but it's in there.

It's straightforward enough - I just have to be strong, that's all. Not weak, not unable, and definitely not incapable. Especially now that we have children. Young kids look up to you so much, innocently expecting that you can solve all the problems in the world - a bit like being their Superman! Of course, at their age they can't see why this might not be so reasonable, but as adults we can. Or so you might expect. In actual fact you start to live this role a little, and begin to believe some of it yourself - at least up to a point. This can enable you to overcome some of your own silly fears, reluctances to do this or that, and face some of the confidence issues that used to hold you back. Now you can push through these barriers because you are doing it for your kids. But still, inside my head, asking for help would be the same as admitting weakness or failure.

Accepting that you can't handle something is difficult enough, more so when it means also admitting that you're not coping. Aside from the macho-male psyche (more on this later), there is also the paranoid mind. Ask for help? Admit to someone what's going on in my head? Uh-oh, they might find out I'm not 'normal'... Ok, so I've always known that I'm not exactly what passes for normal, and don't have a problem with that, but hey, I don't like the idea of strangers knowing. Talking to strangers, especially a medical person of some sort just sounds dangerous. Ask a doctor for help? Tell a doctor what's going on inside my head? They'd probably lock me up! I mean, it's ok just being myself, quirks and all, but how would I prove I'm not mental? I've joked about those things in the past, you know - One Flew Over the Cuckoo's Nest and all of that? Put me in a mental hospital for a day or two and it could be quite a challenge to get out again! But at least then I was joking. Now I am actually worried, really worried about some of the things inside my head.

At the same time, there is also a part of me that is laughing. Laughing at me. Not maliciously, but just at the ludicrous nature of it all - to be honest you really can see the funny side of this. Laugh or cry? Cry or laugh? Maybe both, who knows, it might just be therapeutic...

The bottom line is that when you simply can't get up off the floor by yourself (and believe me, you will know), then no matter how you might feel about it, there is no other option than to swallow your pride and ask for help.

Paul Johnson

3. To Bare One's Soul

So there I was, thinking about going to the doctors and talking to them about everything. In the event, getting my head around the idea proved to be much more difficult than you might have thought. Why? Well, lets be honest here, it's hardly manly is it? *Hello, my name's Paul and I'm weak and pathetic. Please can you help me cope with my little life*? It doesn't seem like a very positive thing to do, it's a bit like having your manhood removed (no, not that bit). Still, in the end, I did decide to go and see my GP...

I wrestled with this in my mind for some time without mentioning it to a soul, because the moment it came up for discussion, I would doubtless be given well meaning advice. And accompanying this advice would be the unspoken pressure to do something about it, to take the next step and to sort it out. All I knew was that I didn't need pressure from anyone, myself included, so instead I waited and pondered on the idea. Although it meant the whole thing stretched out for longer, it also meant that I had sufficient time to think it through properly, to get used to the idea before I had to make any sort of decision. Otherwise I would never have gone.

In truth, I would never have gone to see the doctor for myself, irrespective of how bad things got. Too many feelings of weakness and failure to face - I would rather have crashed and burned than face this for myself. Except I wasn't the only one with a stake in this. My wife, my children, especially my beautiful children - what could they understand of this? How could they make allowances for a 'grown-up' problem that they couldn't possibly comprehend? All they knew was that Daddy kept shouting and yelling, and occasionally smacking. They couldn't understand why sometimes it was ok, but at other times Daddy seemed to have turned into a scary monster. You try remembering the devastation in your child's eyes after they have been screamed at, when they've only committed a relatively minor 'crime', like spilling some juice on the floor. That's what got me to the doctors. The sorry truth is that you can't take back things like that once they've happened. But what you can do is to stop it from happening again (and again and again...).

So there I was, sitting in the waiting room, wondering what on earth I was doing there, and what would all these people think if they knew? It was so tempting to just get up and walk out. I mean, who would know? It's not like anyone was going to drag me back in. Trouble was, I knew that if I walked, then I would never go back, and I was there because of my kids. And my wife, the only person on this whole planet that has ever understood more than one or two parts of me. So I stayed, with the 'noble' thought of *doing it for them.*

A word of advice for the guys out there - ask for an appointment with a female doctor. I didn't, and got a male GP instead. He was sympathetic and said all the right things, but I didn't really open up. I couldn't, not properly. Well, I might have embarrassed myself and got upset or something - you know, made myself look less of a man. And that's just not the done thing, is it...?

So I missed out some of the more delicate details, and settled for outlining my situation in a very matter-of-fact way. It's funny looking back, we could almost have been talking about DIY or the weather.

Mind you, this reluctance to talk is not quite as sad and testosterone-driven as it might sound. There are actually good reasons why I might not want to open up and talk about my problems. For many years I have been a fighter in my approach to life, in that my attitude has always been that I *will* find an answer to whatever problems I have faced, that I *will* find a way through. At times it has been this ingrained belief that has kept me going, and importantly, has also helped me to remain positive through some difficult periods. I might not have known how or when I would find a way around such and such a problem, but I would manage to stay reasonably calm and relaxed, simply because I had every faith that I would find the answer. Persistence, refusal to stop, just keeping going - it is incredible how strong this resilience can be.

And what of the cliché that *men just need to open up and talk about their feelings?* Personally I can't see the point in going over and over old ground. Far from releasing the pressure, this has the opposite effect - stress is actually created by raking through the detail. Chewing over frustrations just seems to bring them closer to the surface, re-running painful experiences like an old video, over and over. Worse, the negativity of it all serves to undermine my resilience, this belief of mine that I will find a way through. Once such a chink is exposed in my armour, then all manner of negative thoughts and feelings seem to find their way in with ease, eating away at my strength, my energy and motivation.

On the other hand, I would have to admit that I would feel uncomfortable, 'soft' even, discussing my current problems and feelings with someone else. Not only someone else, but a stranger? The 'big tough' side of the male psyche can make this very difficult. There are certainly cultural roots to this in the West, probably the world over. I remember as a kid being told to stop crying, stop being a baby. In later years this was compounded by my peers in much the same way, as any sign of weakness was equated with being *some sort of a girl.* I guess this did 'toughen' me up a bit, and started me off with the good old-fashioned British 'stiff upper lip' - take it on the chin, don't let it show. Don't let people see that it bothers you, grit your teeth and just keep smiling, just keep going... There are some good aspects to this, I have to say, but when you read between the lines, it seems that it doesn't actually matter how you feel, or how these things affect you. It becomes apparent that your feelings should be suppressed, and are certainly not there to be talked about! We can all see evidence of this in society today - particularly (though not exclusively) within the male population.

Peer pressure and threats of bullying start at nursery age, something that is particularly obvious with the boys. It is interesting when talking to other parents that the dads usually understand this much better than the mums, presumably on account of having lived through it themselves. Although all kids learn how to assert themselves (and some do it more 'vigorously' than others), there is usually a difference between the boys and girls in terms of the use of, and especially the threat of violence. As a boy I was well aware of bullying long before I knew what it was called. Unspoken threats of violence and domination of peers by intimidation went on all around us from a very early age, whether in a group situation or on a one to one basis. Just a fact of life.

I have to point out that this opinion does not come from having grown up in an especially poor or deprived area, or from having suffered terribly at the hands of bullies. This intimidation was simply an unpleasant but accepted part of life. It still is - I can see exactly the same things going on within my children's schools. Unfortunately this seems to be part of the human condition.

I did suffer from some degree of bullying during my school years. I think most of us do. But this wasn't the stuff that ends in tragedy, plastered across the front of the newspapers. As far as I can tell, my experiences as a teenager were pretty normal. Yes, there were times when I was picked on, made a fool of, left out or ganged up on by the lads I called my friends, but that was only an isolated piece of the picture - the dynamics of a group of teenage lads generally means this is the deal for them all. Looking back there would usually be five or six of us, constantly taking the mickey out of each other, and although it was mostly good natured, at times it could become quite nasty. Sometimes it was spread around, at others one of the lads would be the focus of everyone else's attention. Someone ended up as that day's victim, and we would all join in. Although we might not have liked it when it was our turn, we all loved it when it was someone else and couldn't wait to have a go, stick the metaphorical boot in. It has to be said that this could get very nasty, and the psychological attacks and dominance were far more damaging than anything physical. However, we all did this to each other, willingly and often gleefully, and this passed as our 'norm'.

And so it continues into adulthood. The same intimidating behaviours are used over and over, and although this is often without any real risk of violence, the games of domination and intimidation remain. Many take their place and accept their role, some as bullies, a handful as eternal victims, but most as just occasional victims. Interestingly it can be seen that many of the largest group - the occasional victims - also double up as occasional bullies.

Although this whole cycle is easy to spot, it can be very difficult to break out of. We are conditioned from birth by our experiences, which teach us what to expect, and show us how the world is. In this instance our experiences tell us that the strong will often get away with murder when the teacher, parents or boss isn't looking, or perhaps isn't interested. It doesn't matter when people try to tell us otherwise, as we have all seen thousands of examples of this along the way, in what can often seem to be a terribly unfair world. So we all know the score, we all know how it works. A very negative cycle, and one that can 'keep you in your place' for a lifetime.

A significant number find, as I did, that training in the martial arts can have a dramatic effect on their perception of these events. Assuming that your chosen art/teacher has at least one eye on reality and pressure testing, then your techniques will stand a reasonable chance of delivering the goods in a live situation. Obviously this doesn't happen overnight, a fair amount of blood, sweat and tears are required, as is the willingness to face your own failings along the way. But before long you become increasingly able to deal with the threat of a violent attack. Your confidence in this ability grows, which in turn starts to change your perception, and you find yourself knowing that if violence were to occur, you at last have some chance of dealing with it. As a result, you start to understand how little threat there usually is in front of you, and as the fear reduces, the perceived physical threat starts to diminish and you can at last see the childish ego-driven game of dominance that is behind it all. Now the options start to open up in front of you...

Of course there are exceptions - the violent minority do exist and should not be underestimated. By preparing you for these dangerous individuals however, a good martial art will also equip you for those whose attacks remain psychological. Think about it, if you are prepared for punches, kicks and knife attacks, just how much is a bad attitude or a casual insult going to hurt you? Sticks and stones, you know...?

So now you can face a confrontational situation at work, and ask yourself - just what is this guy going to do/say if I don't go along with him? What exactly is going to happen when I stop this, and politely point out that I am not playing ball, that I going my own way? Answer - the vast majority of the time they will do nothing. Sure they can go sulk, but the intimidation, the subconscious fear of this leading to a violent attack, is now exposed as falsehood.

This breakthrough allows you to start taking control over the invisible threats, the intangible but very real forces that so often hold us back. As a result you can start to take an increasing responsibility for your own life. More on that later, but this breakthrough is a real beginning.

It is noticeable within the martial arts that as students develop and progress to a reasonable level of physical ability, many will also become more gentle in nature. Although this might appear to be a paradox, it is actually pretty straightforward - when you understand violence, and the real implications of violence, you don't want any part of it. Beyond this, as you start to develop some degree of capability in your chosen art, you can also start to discover other 'softer' sides of yourself without feeling vulnerable or exposed. This is perhaps like the Samurai being taught poetry, calligraphy or flower arranging, to compliment the martial studies and become a more complete human being. To become a balanced person, to develop and grow spiritually, and to see this reflected in your everyday life. Something to **really** aspire to.

Back to the doctors, and the follow up appointment a week later. Got a female doctor this time, who opened things up in a different way, and made it easier for me to be honest about things. I did feel vulnerable, but she made that ok, and afterwards I was very glad I had gone through with this. It wasn't just that we didn't have the 'macho male' thing in our way, she also hit the nail right on the head with some of her questions. Where do I get my support? Where is the time for me? Where is the time for us as a couple? (me and my wife, not me and the doctor). If I don't take steps to look after myself, who else will? Who else can? Does my own well-being not hold any priority for me?

Not only were the questions important, but it was also noticeable just how receptive she was. This wasn't your average busy GP, pressed for time and asking the usual questions whilst trying to decide which box you fit into. This was different - a doctor that was really listening, that really did seem to care. She even related some of her advice back to her own family life, and the difficulties that we all face from time to time. Her personal tip was a way to head things off when you can feel the pressure building up. Apparently, you open the back door of your house, and *SCREAM* all of your frustration, at the top of your voice, out into the back garden and beyond. This is supposed to be good for reducing stress, and has been tried and tested by the good doctor for many years. Incidentally, she did warn that it doesn't always make you too popular with the neighbours...

Fast forward a few weeks, I'm back at work, and seem to be managing reasonably well. Things are going better now, at least in the sense of being better than they were. Still a few issues, but I've realised that there aren't any quick fixes, that I can expect to take some time with all of this. And actually, that's ok.

I haven't been back to the doctors, so I guess I'm on my own with it. There is some support at home, but otherwise it's back into the busy lifestyle, standing on my own two feet again. The doctor had mentioned some sort of counselling service that could have supported me, but I wasn't keen, not my cup of tea at all. I didn't try to put up an argument at the time, and she had said it would take months to come through, so I just played along. Anything to avoid the discussion. Appointment over, and I just went home and forgot all about it. Counselling? Me? As if.

A couple of weeks later I received a letter from the counselling people, acknowledging the referral from my GP. The letter was a bit strange really, it had some blurb saying that all problems are rooted in relationships, and that the purpose of counselling was to enable us to talk about our feelings around these relationships, thus getting to the cause of our problems. Would I like to talk about my relationships? In detail? Would I like to talk about how I feel? With a stranger? I would rather stick pins in my eyes, thank you very much, or try to dig my heart out with a spoon... Oh yeah, great - thanks for offering, but it's *really* not for me...

It seemed to me as if they were prejudging the situation before they had even met me. I'm not stupid - I know that professionals sometimes think in very broad-brush terms, but still... if they had already decided that my problems were rooted in my relationships, then I definitely wasn't going. Call me old fashioned, but I rather thought it would be nice if someone were to listen to me before they decide what's wrong. You know, actually meet me, and hear what

I've got to say first? Understand what I think, how I feel? Stupid of me, I know. Anyhow, mind made up, I read the rest of the letter, which said that I would need to give them a call if I wanted to go on the waiting list. Needless to say, I didn't bother, thinking that was the end of it. But I was wrong.

Another couple of weeks on, and I'm looking in amazement at a letter from these people, giving a time and date for my appointment with a Counsellor. Hello, what's going on here? I don't remember making that call...

But an appointment has been made, somehow. It actually exists. I'm staring at the letter, wondering. The letter stares back, daring me. Not sure what to do - I feel like a rabbit caught in the headlights. I know that I don't want to go. I know why I don't want to go. Still, here I am wondering - I mean, I'm not a hundred percent yet, far from it if I'm honest. What I've got here is someone offering help, and I'm not completely certain that an instant refusal is in my best interests. Ok, so the initial letter was off-putting, but I don't really know what it is that these people do, or what might happen in a counselling session. My experiences in the martial arts have taught me that sometimes you need to step forward into discomfort. That if you want a different outcome, then you have to do something different. Hmm, I'm really not sure about this, but sometimes you have to put opinions, presumptions and personal preferences to one side and dive right in. Only then are you really in a position to judge if something works for you.

So I pick up the phone, and ring the number. It's a bit surreal, talking to the receptionist, all along thinking that this doesn't make sense for me, this isn't the sort of thing I do... The lady on the phone makes it all feel OK, and before you know it I have confirmed my appointment. Once I've been to the first session, I will officially be a fucked up individual who is undergoing counselling. Not sure I like the sound of that.

The day comes at last, and I arrive a bit flustered, almost late. I've belted back from a really busy morning at work, driving well over the speed limit most of the way. Not ideal preparation. Still, on the plus side it means I haven't given it too much thought, which must be a good thing... Get inside, take a seat, and a few minutes later I'm in with the Counsellor. It's all a bit strange, because it's suddenly quite hard to explain why I'm here. Harder still to know how to summarise everything, to give a concise version of events that fits into a forty minute session, and know that I've remembered to mention all of the relevant bits... I mean, now that I'm here and have opened up a bit, I seem to be feeling alright about talking, so it would be better if we had several hours. At least then we could go through from start to finish, but this? This is strange. It's also quite surreal to be talking about things that are normally kept under wraps, to have them out in the open as if this were a normal everyday conversation. Anyway, we get through to the end of the first session, and it wasn't too bad. I still wasn't sure about signing up for six weeks, but to be fair, there was never any pressure from their side.

Although I wasn't certain what I'd actually gained from the session, one or two comments stayed in my head afterwards, and I found myself thinking a little differently. For example, the Counsellor had suggested that I seem to be carrying a great deal of frustration. Hmmm, lots of possible reasons, probably some truth in most of them, but I started to ask myself if these were merely symptoms, if perhaps I hadn't yet realised what the underlying cause was. I will pick up on that in a later chapter, however for the moment it is sufficient to say that the sessions I attended did stimulate a lot of thought, and the benefits of going (which far outweighed my reluctance) were mainly realised in the days that followed each appointment.

Although the whole counselling experience is not one that I had ever expected to have, I would certainly recommend it - it's surprising just how accurately someone on the outside can cut right through to the heart of an issue. Usually because you're just too close to see it for yourself. I wouldn't worry about different styles, or any myths or stories you might have heard about counselling. After all, different approaches will always suit different people.

The important thing to consider is that there are well-trained people out there, who are prepared to listen and help you at a time when you really need the support. Is it the right way forward for you?

Well, if you don't go along, and do so with an open mind, then you will never know. But this has to be worth a shot - after all, it might just be the thing that helps turn your life around.

STARTING TO UNDERSTAND

Paul Johnson

4. The Main Cause Of Anxiety

Over the weeks that followed, I began to realise that a great deal of the discomfort and anxiety in my life is actually caused by (guess who?) myself. For example, one of my kids has a medical appointment this week at the local hospital. It's something beyond the normal routine stuff, so both myself and my wife need to be there. As much for each other as for the kids. As it happens, our appointment clashes with an major training event at work, so I can't possibly go - I mean, this event is really important, to do with legal issues that will affect how we work in the future. Worse still, it follows on from a previous event that I missed for similar reasons. If it wasn't for missing the last one, then maybe, but now? I mean, how would it look? I can't miss this, I'd never get up to speed getting the information second hand from someone else - besides there are expectations you know, professional standards to be upheld. It's part of the job, and I can't not do my job properly, I mean, it's what I get paid for, I can't possibly miss this and be unprofessional and uninformed and look bad and feel bad and... ARRRGGGHHH!!

Believe me, I really do wish that I was making this up to illustrate a point. But I'm not. After spinning out of control for some time, I finally caught hold of myself, and the conversation inside my head went something like this:

What is this about?

My family's well-being.

Is that not the most important thing in the world?

Well, yes, but...

How much does your wife need you on this day?

Hmm, quite a lot I suppose.

And how important is that?

Well obviously it's important, but...

And what about work - would your colleagues really object?

I don't suppose they would really...

Your boss, would she really be difficult?

Well, no, I guess not..

What would she say if you talked to her about this 'dilemma'?

Errm, she would probably tell me to stop being daft and go look after my kids.

And catching up afterwards? Remember, the all-important legal stuff?

Hmm, I suppose I could get this from someone. From a few people, come to think of it.

OK, so your kids need you, your wife needs you, and these are the most important things in the world, right?

Yeah...

And your workmates and boss will understand, no real harm will be done, and you can catch up with whatever you miss?

Yeah...

So you know what to do?

Yes.

And do you feel stupid now?

Errm, yes.

Do you think all this grief could have been avoided?

Choose Life

Yes, I guess so...

Do you know where this all came from?

Well - no, not really.

It came from you - all of the stress and upset was avoidable. You created it by allowing your thoughts to spiral downwards. Worse still it was only a perceived problem, which in reality will take no more than a quick phone call to resolve. The rest is all your own creation - completely unnecessary and entirely avoidable.

Oh.

Time to start doing things differently, and stop this nonsense.

But how?

By taking a step back - try to look at things as if you were advising a friend, see things in their proper perspective. And other times just stop thinking. Be quiet, keep your thoughts still and *feel* for the proper flow of things.

Different people create stress and anxiety for themselves in different ways - this can be illustrated by looking at a couple of my colleagues from work, Richard and Keith, two guys that I worked alongside a few years ago (I have changed their names, but everything else is true to life). By way of introduction, they are in their late thirties-early forties, and both are experienced in their field. They have very different natures, each with self-evident strengths and weaknesses, but both seem to get the job done.

Richard is a guy that is clearly dedicated and cares about the role. He feels the weight of responsibility a bit too heavily at times, but strives to do the right thing and usually delivers the goods. And if he doesn't, then I know that it isn't for the want of trying. If things do go wrong, then he will hold his hands up and be honest, and sort it out quickly afterwards. This guy takes it personally, and you know that it is all honest, all straight from the heart. If something has gone awry, he will go away and brood, and this will often trouble him for a while. I know that's not always good, but you can be sure he will learn from it, and come through it as a more capable person for the experience. A recent development however is that he went off sick for a couple of weeks with stress, so now we need to keep on eye on him, and give him some support when he starts taking too much on. But otherwise, what a star - I wish we had more like him.

Keith is a different kettle of fish entirely, and is one I have always suspected of being a bit lazy. He is entirely likeable, and good fun to have around - a born entertainer. His work seems to stand up to scrutiny, although I have to say it's never been under the microscope. I know something isn't right though. The biggest giveaway is that he's just too laid back - I'm not knocking it as an approach, to be honest I'm usually fairly relaxed myself and try to take it all with a sense of humour. But this feels different, like he's taking the mickey. Those around him will quietly voice the same opinion - when everyone else is always busy, always on the go, this guy never seems to break a sweat. You know, I've been around a while, seen it all before - you can't fool me so easily. It isn't difficult to figure that he is just going through the motions without any real commitment. Maybe he's off-loading work elsewhere, or just being clever about the jobs he does, making sure they're the ones least likely to be noticed. On the odd occasion when they are, he is quick to acknowledge any faults and apologise, saying it was an oversight. Well, we all like someone who is honest about their mistakes, right? Hmmm - other people might buy it, but not me. Not from him.

In addition, I know that despite the façade of happy-go-lucky, Keith is far from content with his lot. Sure, he makes the best of it, gets through with a mask of humour and sarcasm, but on the odd occasions when no-one else has been around, he has actually dropped this front. Just a couple of times, but when he loses the attitude and opens up a bit, it's very clear that he is not at all satisfied with his life. Beneath the surface, it seems that he wonders if this is all that there is, and secretly longs for more depth, more substance to his life. It's well hidden from view for the most part, but it's there.

Choose Life

I was talking with another colleague recently, who also has a dim view of Keith's approach, and who would love to see him slip and get caught out. During this conversation I started to wonder whether everything is really as it seems, as we have all assumed.

Look again at Richard - yes, he's dependable, full of enthusiasm, and utterly reliable. Yes, he will make sure the job is done. But is that really such a good thing? From his employer's point of view then perhaps it is, but let's take a wider perspective for a moment. This is making him ill, he's taking work so seriously that it is having an impact on his health. The guy has been off with stress - something I now understand, something I now have very different views on.

What about the effect on his family - it's not like this is a single guy that can go home and chill out, he's married with a couple of kids. I know his wife works full-time and isn't very supportive either, so life must be pretty hectic at home. We can only guess at the impact that Richard's stress levels are having on his home-life (because us blokes don't talk about sissy stuff like that), but it isn't likely to be good. Besides, why is he taking too much on board? Is this because the company are taking advantage of his good nature? Is it because he struggles to make good use of his time, doesn't understand how to prioritise? Perhaps he finds it hard to say 'no', and allows others to off-load work onto him? Just think, a minute ago Richard was the ideal worker, but now you have to wonder...

And what about our friend Keith? From a different perspective, perhaps things aren't as bad as they seem. I mean, this is a guy that is keeping on top of his job, no obvious problems, and certainly no complaints. The fact that he doesn't take issues home with him and can switch off from the demands of the job, this must actually make his home life less fraught. Not causing grief at home, not making him ill either? Has to be a positive in the wider scheme of things. What else - he seems to make it look easy? Well, perhaps his approach makes it easier. Perhaps this is not a cover for someone slacking, but just the fact that you can be more productive if you're fairly relaxed and happy rather than strung out and ready to snap. Perhaps it is beneficial to care a little bit less about your job, in fact you might take the view that you could become more effective, a better worker even, as a result of being less bothered...

Confused? So am I.

Bottom line is that the guy who is trying his hardest to do the right thing, to be a good person, is definitely building his own levels of stress and anxiety. Richard is creating much of his own pain through his approach to life, and yes, actually he could learn something from Keith, however unpalatable it might seem at face value. However, although some of Keith strategies are worth using, his selfish intentions, poor engagement and lack of motivation are not a recipe for a fulfilling life.

On balance I would say that neither of these guys are lined up for any degree of happiness or contentment, let alone pushing forward their own growth or development. Personally, I have 'been' both of these guys at different stages in my life, and neither were sustainable positions for me. My advice to Keith would be to stop being so selfish in his approach, as this will always be empty and unfulfilling in the end. He should try taking a greater responsibility and give more to others, in terms of time, help and kindness. I would also explain this as being ultimately selfish, as one of the main goals here is to discover a more fulfilling life for yourself. As contradictory as this might sound, it could just appeal to Keith's nature, and in doing so help him to find a different way, a better way.

My advice to Richard would be to give himself a pat on the back for his honesty, commitment and enthusiasm. I would also point out the errors of his ways, and that he has to start balancing this out by looking after himself. After all, how do you continue to serve others, be a good father or partner, deliver a good service at work or in the community - how can you sustain this in the longer term if you don't take the time to look after yourself? To do this, he needs to take a leaf out of others' books, and learn how to avoid taking work home, whether literally or mentally. Learn how to take a step back in order to maintain a more balanced and happy life. Ironically he will find himself more productive for doing so.

Vitally for Richard, he must hang on to the things he's got right thus far, and make sure he maintains this integrity and honesty throughout any changes - this is important if he is to grow and find balance as a person. It can be a difficult process at times, but hey, if it was easy then everyone would be doing it! When he starts to work towards this, Richard will find that he is more upbeat and positive, has more energy and feels altogether healthier. He should even find some of the old buzz again, and what could be better than that?

Because of his tendency to put everyone else first, Richard may well feel that to take a less 'full-on' approach would be selfish. A key point in turning his thinking around is to help him to see this as something he should really do for others. That by putting himself first occasionally he will be better placed to continue to serve and support those around him.

These guys might or might not take this on board, but clearly they are both causing much of the stress, anxiety and discomfort in their lives. Understanding this is the first step, and many simply don't. Taking responsibility for your own life is the second step, and the majority won't.

But you can.

5. Whose Responsibility Is It Anyway?

A few years ago, a book that I was reading made the point that everything in your life is actually your own responsibility, even (or perhaps especially) if others are treating you badly. I think the example used was an abusive boss at work, and the message was that in this situation you would have to take action to help yourself. That might be talking to colleagues, talking to your boss, or even his/her boss if necessary. If that didn't work then you might consider trying to arrange a transfer, or if all else failed, look for another job. But the responsibility for your life belongs to you, and you alone.

I found this mind blowing - so simple, but what a revelation! And totally empowering. I have kept this in mind ever since, and can certainly say that it changed my outlook on life, particularly on how I react to the seemingly unreasonable actions of others. Several years on (it can take me a while), I eventually realised that I had only grasped half of the lesson, and that it goes far deeper than just taking responsibility for your actions. How about taking responsibility for your **thoughts too**...?

The first thing to recognise about your thoughts, is that they don't exist anywhere except inside your head. Stating the obvious maybe, but think about it - suppose you might feel angry towards your partner because of something they have said, or perhaps you feel that they don't listen to you, don't value your opinion. You then spend the next hour or two getting more and more worked up, running it over and over in your mind, adding a little more self-righteousness each time around until you're all revved up and ready to go. Then when your partner comes in, you are going to let them have it, no matter what they do or say. You won't be thinking straight, and you certainly won't be listening. You will simply explode like a cork from a bottle, with all that self-righteous anger, pent-up frustration from the crap week you've had, and all the other negatives in your system at that moment. All of it - WHAM - out it comes.

There's no need for a hypothetical situation here - it would be fair to say that we've been around this particular loop a good few times.

What usually happens is that I end up looking like the bad guy, even if I'd started out with right on my side (which I had, at least twice). Anyhow, the last time this started to build up, I actually managed to get in before the big explosion. I could see it coming, feel myself getting less tolerant and more pointedly sarcastic with each moment that passed. Time to go, quick before I said something really damaging - grabbed the dog lead (and the dog), and out of the house. Whew!

My intention was just to get out, avoid the big shouting match and give myself a few minutes to calm down. Off I went, dragging the dog down the road, round the corner and off towards the park. I was twice round the cricket pitch before realising that I was route-marching, still running it all through my head, re-fighting the battle over and over again. At this point I tried to relax, slow things down, looking for the proper flow of things, but couldn't seem to find it. Realising that I was all tense, I deliberately relaxed everything physically. Then everything mentally. Trying to let the negative thoughts go in the breeze, but not quite managing it. So I stopped.

It's very rare that I actually stop, and do nothing. Busy life, lots of running around, and always something to do next. Never stop until it's late, then collapse for an hour in front of the telly before bed. Anyway, there I was in the middle of the local park at 10pm, unable to see anything in the pitch blackness other than the silhouettes of a few trees and houses. Standing. Just standing, no thoughts, no nothing. Just standing. An age passed, and then the stress and tension started to fall away. I might have only been still for a minute or two, but somehow all sense of time had gone - it could have been hours. The confusion and emotions started to clear, just enough to see which thoughts were real and valid, and which weren't. So I felt a bit better, and thought about walking on. But I didn't. This time I stayed put. I've dabbled with some bits & bobs of meditation before, nothing serious, but I have played with some of the basics. So I decided to stay where I was, still standing in the darkness of the park, and think my situation through. Not force it through with the analytical side of my head, but let if float through, contemplate things, a bit like the meditation stuff.

Choose Life

...... so.................. why is my wife reacting to me in this way? .... oh yeah, I remember .... she's had an especially tough day today............... I knew that............ hmm, not sure how I managed to forget that earlier............ come to think of it, she actually needed my support............ she did seem a bit abrasive though............ mind you, hardly surprising given the difficult day she's had today............

Alone in the darkness, it finally dawned on me that at the precise moment my wife needed some love and support, I had managed to shout at her, get myself feeling all hurt and defensive, and then buggered off up the park with the dog! And what did I feel at this point of revelation? Love. Compassion. Ok, ok, maybe a tinge of guilt as well... I put the dog back on the lead and headed off home to apologise and try to make things right. All along thinking *this didn't need to have happened.*

The point of that story? Well, although it can seem complicated when you try to apply these ideas and principles to real life, it should actually be pretty straight forward. It only becomes complicated when our emotions kick in, and then we often struggle to see which way is up. Also, I seem to have an unerring ability to say the wrong things, to instinctively press the wrong buttons, often making things far, far worse than they ever needed to be. Something to do with being male, or so I'm told...

A page or two back I stated that thoughts and emotions don't exist anywhere except inside your head - this is true, but only for as long as the thoughts stay there. Once you allow this to influence your actions, behaviours or moods, then it becomes part of reality, and starts to impact on other people. In the example above, I didn't get a grip quickly enough to prevent any damage from being done, but I did realise before it got out of hand.

A key point here is to understand that you can stop these thoughts before they take on a life of their own, before they grow into something uncontrollable. You can stop them in their tracks and create an alternative outcome. Tell yourself - *I'm not having this, these are only thoughts. They might be uncomfortable but they're not real, they only exist in my head, and I will not be dictated to. I'm*

*going to make my own choices, instead of feeling like I'm acting out
a scripted part where the future seems to have already been decided
by apparently inevitable choices.*

There are frequently times when this opportunity comes well within
your grasp, and I will come back to this a little further on. For the
moment though, just contemplate the possibilities here, the options
that open up. The idea of taking responsibility for yourself in **every**
way, in both your thoughts and deeds, is both daunting and
exhilarating. Scary in some ways, but can you imagine the potential
freedom, the potential of your creativity, in fact the potential of your
whole life, if you can just put this into practice?

Another perspective on taking responsibility can be seen by looking
at the concepts of Yin and Yang. Seemingly different opinions and
definitions provide some degree of confusion, however, instead of
thinking of these as just terms of contradictory or opposing views,
we need to consider Yin and Yang at different levels of
understanding. At a basic level, they can indeed mean opposites or
polarities, such as light and dark, hard and soft, positive and
negative, male and female and so on. Nothing wrong with this,
however the Yin and Yang concept can help us to understand
something more about the world we live in, rather than just being a
useful way of describing opposites.

At a deeper level, we start to see that although complete opposites
may seem to exist, in truth a given situation is never totally one
thing or the other. If we look closely at something that is usually
thought of as negative, there is always an element of positive in
there as well. It might be a very small element, but it is there if you
look closely. It may be no more than the spark of potential for a
positive outcome, but there is a 'silver lining' to be found, for those
that are minded to look. This holds true for almost all situations.
Bear in mind there are few things in life that are truly black or
white, but instead many, many different shades of grey.

Keeping this in mind, look at the circular black & white
representation of the Yin and Yang concept. You can see that the
black swirls into the white, and the white into the black.

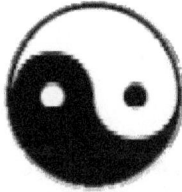

However, there is also a small area of black within the white area, and vice versa. This is said to represent how everything contains the seed of its opposite within it, and is symbolic of how all things contain both Yin and Yang.

A third version of events sees us considering the original written characters for Yin and Yang. The symbol for Yang, taken in the most literal way, is said to have meant 'the light side of the mountain, bright, warm and sunny'. By contrast, the symbol for Yin meant the 'dark side of the mountain, shaded, cold and wet'. With this in mind, you can see that we are no longer looking at opposites - in fact we are now looking at different views of the same thing. Different perceptions of the same mountain.

Like many of us, I used to think - *yeah, I've heard this sort of thing before, I get the general picture, got the gist of it.* Although this was true in one sense, I would still struggle to find any real practical use for these ideas - this frustration seems to accompany many 'mystical' teachings from the East. The significance (or at least one significance) of these concepts finally came to me on a family day out. Picture the scene - it's Saturday morning, just had a big argument with my wife, wasn't even sure what it was about at the time. We're heading south on the motorway to visit the in-laws, an hour and a half drive ahead of us. The atmosphere is so tense that you could grate cheese on it and the kids are being little sods in the back of the car, shouting, yelling, fighting, and generally winding me up. It's hot, the sun is blazing through the windscreen, and I'm getting uncomfortable. I haven't got a drink, and can already feel the beginnings of a headache coming on. The car is filled with unspoken tension, I'm ready to start shouting at the kids, and this is setting the tone for the whole day. Maybe even the whole weekend.

Not good.

As the minutes pass by in stony silence, I start thinking about mountains, and different perceptions. Start to think that maybe if I tried, my current situation might, just might seem different. Perhaps I should try to take myself out of the situation, and see things more objectively...

Now that I have stopped to think, I can see it's actually a beautiful day - the sun is shining, and it's pretty warm for a March weekend. The kids are playing in the back of the car, just messing about and having fun. Not really fighting, just acting their ages and being noisy with it, enjoying each others' company. Then I look outside, away from the three lanes of tarmac. Beautiful green fields and lush countryside stretch for miles on both sides. I can see fields, wooded areas, occasional houses and farm buildings - the things you wouldn't usually notice, because you're simply not looking. This was exactly the same journey, just seen from a different perspective.

I started to understand that the way we view our situation has a huge influence on how we interact with it. This will impact on our actions, moods and feelings, and in turn have a knock-on effect on those around us, and their actions, moods and so on. At this point you realise that although you are never in complete control of a situation, you can choose to steer in this direction or that. Importantly, the situation is not in control of you - you are not destined to have a crap day, and the outcome is not predetermined. Instead you have choices in front of you.

With this, I lost the option to make excuses, and found I had responsibility instead. The fact is that it is no else's fault, that it's down to you as an individual - you alone can decide which way your day/week/life goes. Let's be clear here, I'm not saying it's easy, but I am saying you can decide to choose a different path if you wish.

Choose Life

At the end of the day, the most important thing is that we are happy in our lives. For me, finding I have some influence over areas that I previously thought were out of my control has been liberating. It's perhaps a little scary as well, because the buck stops with me now, but it comes with a sense of freedom, a definite feeling that nothing will ever be quite the same again. There is a huge amount of potential here, and all of it is positive.

And as for my journey on that day? Well, the mood did change as we continued down the motorway, and we got back on track again. This shift in perspective helped to divert what was starting to look like a very grim day. OK it wasn't perfect, but then we're all human, and for me this was a beginning. I still have much work and practice to do in this area, but at least I now understand that I no longer have any excuses

So, not only is the responsibility yours, but you also know what to do. Next time things are looking bad, give it a go - take a look at the other side of the mountain. You'll find the sun is usually shining...

Paul Johnson

6. The Cop-out

I keep coming across the story of the five blind men who were asked to describe an elephant - this originated from a parable-type story within Hinduism, although it has been adapted over recent years for use in a variety of arenas. The story tells that the elephant was standing in front of the five men, and they were each asked to describe what they could feel. The first had hold of the trunk, the second had a tusk, the third had an ear, the fourth had a leg, and the fifth had the tail. Despite the fact they all described in detail what it was they had hold of, accurately and succinctly, not one of them had any idea what an elephant looked like. The point of course, is that none of them could 'see' the whole picture. The same can be said for the vast majority of the world's large-scale organised religions. Most can be seen to have genuine spiritual teachings at their heart, but have a tendency to focus on 'this' or 'that' aspect, rather than the essence of the teachings. This focus on detail leads to a narrowing of perspective, and they often lose their view of the bigger picture along the way. The whole elephant, if you like.

So it is with many of the self-help books that are available. When you go and look in bookshops or on the Internet, you will be amazed. There are books to help guide you through every conceivable part of life, the whole mind, body and spirit thing is there, spread across a few shelves. A wealth of information from across the world, giving countless techniques, practices and disciplines for us to choose from. So many in fact, that it can become a nightmare for the seeker on the path - how do you know where to look, what to try, how these techniques might gel together or whether they actually conflict with one another? The focus of self-help books are often technique based - I guess that is what most of the general public are looking for when they spend their hard-earned on such a book. If I'm to part with my £9.99 (or often more) then what I want is a step by step guide, an easy 'how-to' book that will provide methods I can easily apply to my life, and in doing so, sort out all of the problems that led me here in the first place. Over simplifying? Well, maybe… but only a little.

Irrespective of the reasons why, what we often get are books full of 'helpful' techniques, which is great if you are lucky enough to hit upon one that really does work for you. Of course there are benefits to looking at techniques and methods that might be useful, and there are inevitably a few within these pages. When we adopt such a technique to help us identify the (apparent) causes of our stress and anxiety, or to help us to relax our over-stimulated minds after a long day at work, this has to be a step in the right direction. A definite positive. However, we often continue to miss the bigger picture - we're looking so hard at the details that we don't see the bloody great elephant that is standing right in front of us!

By focussing on techniques and missing the overall picture, this also provides an opt-out clause, a built-in excuse to cop-out. *Oh no, that technique wouldn't work for me. No, this method doesn't fit into my lifestyle. No, I don't quite understand what they're getting at...* Sound familiar at all? Maybe some things are difficult to understand, maybe some genuinely wouldn't be right for you or your lifestyle, but there is another side to this. Finding the right path will involve work and effort, and usually an acknowledgement of having been wrong in some of your thoughts and actions to date. We are often not ready to face this, perhaps preferring to wallow in our situation a little longer before facing the pain that we associate with taking responsibility for ourselves. *You mean you actually expect me to do something?!* It is at this point that the excuses will flow, and within a book full of specific techniques and fixed disciplines, it becomes all too easy to opt out.

Ian (a friend of mine) had a similar experience a few weeks ago, and was reading an article which related closely to a personal problem that he had been struggling with for a while. In Ian's case he wasn't in denial - he understood only too well how the advice related to his situation, but was extremely uncomfortable because it was just too close to home. It didn't have the 'feel-good' factor about it, the advice wasn't wrapped up and disguised by fancy language or the author's need to avoid upsetting anyone. It was written in plain language, cut through the crap and got right down to the heart of the matter. As a result, my friend started to realise that aside from being uncomfortably close to home, this was leading towards him having to face up to one or two truths, and take some sort of action. Or to put it another way, to take responsibility. He felt that this was more than he could handle at that moment in time, and simply put the article down. Unfortunately he couldn't bring himself to pick it back up - a real shame when it was something that might really have helped his situation. All is not lost however, as Ian is an intelligent guy, and although he bottled out on that occasion, he knows it. Hopefully when he is feeling a little stronger, then Ian will pick up the article again, and carry on where he left off.

Back to the books full of various techniques - we go on to finish the last chapter, wisely nodding our heads at the good advice within. We might even have picked out a long list of suggestions and changes that we want to make, but we keep the list inside our head. Then we get on with our lives, having failed to do anything different as a result. We reduce this book, with its enormous life changing potential, to be nothing more than an 'interesting read'.

Others will at least try, but when counter-balancing years of drudgery, we have a tendency to overdo it, and often by identifying a dozen or more action points that we need to address. We write them down, not realising that this exhaustive list, however positive our intentions, is simply overwhelming. And as a result, not sustainable. I will come back to the subject of goal setting in a later chapter, but the important thing here is to accept there is a balance to be found, and maintained. In this context, the balance is between doing too little, and attempting to do too much. There is no rule to say that we can't have occasional bursts of development, however in the main our progress needs to be at a pace that is sustainable. A step a day, every day, and you will soon find that you have travelled a surprising distance. And if some days you find that you feel like running ahead a little, so much the better. On other days, just walk.

As for the books overflowing with advice - sure, take a look, after all there are some wonderful ideas out there. Just be sure that you pick out the ones that seem right for you, and avoid the temptation to try everything at once. Many of these things are just different approaches to the same goal, and you only need to find one or two that are right for you.

Above all else, you must be honest with yourself, and remember that the responsibility is yours. Sure, some techniques will help along the way, but without the solid foundation of self-honesty, the techniques themselves are little more than sticking plasters. And if you do 'fail', if you do cop-out - then what? Accept the experience as a step towards your goal, pick yourself up, dust yourself down and keep going. Just keep going.

It may not sound too revolutionary to say that this is the answer, but I am reminded of a conversation I once had with an experienced martial arts instructor. He asked if I knew the difference between those that gained the much desired black belt, and those that fell by the wayside? My answer was nothing if not predictable - *dedication, spirit, commitment, a great love of the art, discipline.* This wasn't exactly wrong, but his answer was much simpler. He told me that the students who managed to earn a black belt were simply the ones that kept turning up each week. And it is true - whether you fall foul of the negative voice inside your head, whether you trip and stumble along the path - refusing to give up and simply keeping going is a sure-fire way to achieve your goals.

7. The 'Proper' Flow Of Things

I began delving into the mysteries of the martial arts some years ago, and in addition to the hours on the mat, I have also spent a good deal of time studying some of the accompanying philosophies. At times this has been closely tied to the physical training, and at others more concerned with the application of martial wisdom in its widest sense. Some degree of development on the physical level was of course inevitable, but surprisingly there has been more growth in the psychological and spiritual realms. The most fascinating areas are the ones that lie somewhere in-between, those that aren't so easy to define, or neatly classify as being 'this' or 'that'.

Hands-on training in the dojo varies from the immediacy of a confrontation or attack through to the longer-term development of principles, and the fluidity of movement and thought. Within this are exercises in sensitivity training, a few of which look at the concept of picking up the 'killing intention' of an attacker, rather than waiting for a physical assault. This intention is given out subconsciously by virtually all animals at the point of attacking, when they intend to seriously harm or kill their prey. You can see this in nature fairly readily, but it is also evident on CCTV footage of violent assaults in this, our 'civilised' society. The idea of the sensitivity training is that we can pick up on this intention, much the same as animals do when preyed upon in the wild. Whether on the plains of Africa or around the urban inner cities closer to home, an instinctive sensitivity to our attacker's intentions can be the difference between life and death. Our work in the dojo was not a product of concentrated focus, instead it had more to do with relaxing, letting go and just *feeling* the intentions of your would-be attacker. Sounds unlikely? I thought so...

We had some fun playing with this at first, although the most difficult part was trying to generate a genuine feeling of bad intention, when playing the role of attacker. After a while, I found that when 'defending', my body was starting to move itself out of the way of the unseen attacks. No-one was more surprised than myself, as I had made no conscious thoughts or decisions, and the conditions were such that I couldn't see or hear anything to give the attack away. No clues, nothing to react to. This was somewhere beyond cause and effect thinking *(if he does this, I'll do that),* somewhere simpler, someplace more in tune with the natural world. It is difficult to describe as this is a feeling, an instinctive knowledge of some impending discomfort, of something being wrong. A feeling that that you need to move, only to find that you have moved already. To be more precise, my body had moved itself out of the way. I was subconsciously picking up on the intention to cause me harm, which my training partner was starting to give out a second or so before beginning his attack, and was moved by something other than my own conscious self. No decision, no thought - my body simply moved itself without waiting for the rational mind to get involved.

This experience was both moving and bewildering, and gave me first hand proof that such things are indeed possible. It led me to challenge some of my beliefs and assumptions about the universe in which we live, and was enough to finally suspend my disbelief, my deep-rooted scepticism of those things that can't be seen or measured. Still, as incredible as this 'sensing of intention' may seem, it has also been said that it is only the beginning. After all, not everything that could cause you harm will have a killing intention - for example, a dead branch falling out of a tree, a flood, or some other natural event or disaster. So, the next steps are to strive towards feeling the flow of energy, and understanding the intentions of the universe. I know how unlikely this is starting to sound, but bear with me, as this was to have a major impact on my everyday life.

Until recently, my own experiences around this broader idea of feeling the flow of energy of the universe were real, but, well... kind of trivial. For example, when I was relaxed and 'in tune' with things, I might feel a strong urge to take a different route to work as I approached a junction or crossroads. When I followed this feeling, I would get a good run to work, with little sign of the morning rush-hour. If however, I ignored it, I would invariably hit heavy traffic and arrive late. Not just once or twice, this started to happen on a regular basis.

Choose Life

The same goes for parking - I first saw this when my wife was driving. She's usually pretty laid back, and would drive right up to the front of a very busy car park, ignoring my stressed out pleas to *take that space, it's as good as we'll get, quick or we'll lose it!* She would calmly cruise right to the very front, and pull into the space that was waiting for her. It was as if she somehow knew it would be there. Again, this sounds unlikely, but it has happened time and time again - far too often to dismiss as coincidence. This now gets referred to (laughingly) as 'Zen Parking'!

Of course if I **try** to pick up the right feeling as I approach the traffic lights, it doesn't work. If I **try** to arrive at an empty parking space, it simply isn't there. You can't force this, you can't make it happen. In fact the harder you try, the further away you get. So instead, you allow yourself to become receptive to these feelings or energies by simply slowing down and letting go, both physically and mentally.

This happened quite a few times, and was quite fascinating for a while. However, I eventually came to the conclusion that this wasn't quite life changing stuff, pushed it to the 'unexplained bits and pieces' part of my mind, and let it be.

A few weeks after these experiences we had bought a puppy, thinking that it would be great for the kids to have a pet to look after. This inevitably meant that I became the 'lucky' person who got to take it for a walk every morning and night. I began to enjoy the fresh air and the gentle exercise, and found myself looking forward to it. Whether this was 7am in the rain, or 11pm in the dark, it didn't matter. I began to use the time to slow my mind from the rush of daily living, and to practise breathing techniques. A walking meditation of sorts, pausing regularly to stand quietly among the trees, just breathing and feeling.

After five minutes or so of walking in a morning, the birds would start to sing to me. Absolutely amazing. What's more, this would happen every morning, as if the birds were greeting me - what a glorious feeling! Of course, they were really singing all the time, but it took me this long to slow down my over-stimulated brain, and actually notice. It still takes a few minutes sometimes, but now I smile when the birds 'start' to sing, as I recognise what this means - that I have relaxed properly.

After a couple of weeks of this 'walking meditation', I started to experience a very strange feeling. This was like the flow and ebb of the sea, like my mind was being gently pulled by an unseen tide, backwards and forwards. A rhythm, a pulse, a definite 'feeling', and one which grew in strength over the days that followed. What became intriguing was the consistency of this feeling, and how it would only happen when I slowed down, opened my senses and tuned in to the world around me. I remember this once being described by someone as *slowing down to the speed of life*, and this deliberate effort to open my senses soon became something of a daily game. Whenever I realised that I was rushing or stressed, I would consciously slow down and look for this feeling. And find it.

Admittedly, I was a little bewildered by the fact I had no idea what this was, but I felt certain that 'it' was connected with nature, and was a real find, a treasure of some sort. I was also quite amused by the fact I knew there were very few people aside from my wife that I could actually discuss this with. I am very lucky, as she is probably the most open-minded person I have ever met, but what about the rest of my family and friends? They've always known me to be a bit strange, but this would be beyond the pale for most of them...

Around this time I had a peculiar experience that was to have a dramatic impact on my life. I was about to nip up to the local shops (domestically orientated, as ever), when I had a very strong feeling that I shouldn't go, as if this was something I *really* shouldn't do. Nah, I told myself, don't be silly, and shrugged it off. But the feeling persisted. My wife had gone out earlier with the kids, and I thought maybe it's just that she's already bought the same stuff, we connect like this sometimes. Oh well, into the car - more strong feelings, not good. I drove the half mile to the shops, parked up and got out. Same feelings, and just as strong. I was on red alert at this stage, thinking that I might run into a mugger, a gang or some other dangerous situation - after all there could be something to this. Nothing happened. Went to a second shop, still with the same feelings and alertness, but still nothing. Got back in the car and set off home, thinking 'how strange', and dismissing it all as fanciful nonsense. I mean, I haven't got a track record of paranoia, but who knows...?

A hundred yards from home, and suddenly the brake lights came on in front of me. I just managed to stop in time, when BANG, something hit me from behind. Looked in the mirror - nothing. Looked again, still nothing. I went to get out of the car, and nearly jumped out of my skin to see a guy in a motorbike helmet lying on the road! Right there, next to the drivers door! He had hit my back end and been thrown right over to land near the front of the car. As it turned out, this guy was all right other than being black and blue (although we did have some shenanigans around the insurance, but that's a different story). Bottom line of this? Well, there was no real harm done, but it made me think again about things…

I know that when people tell unlikely tales such as this, it's easier (and safer) just to write it off as coincidence, to mentally shrug your shoulders and forget about it. Better than challenging your own beliefs and understanding of the universe, I mean, hey - who wants a hard life after all? But when it happens to you, it's different. When it happens to you, it is undeniably real. I knew, *absolutely knew* from the start that I shouldn't be going out in the car, and the only thing I did wrong was to ignore those feelings. Why? Simply because my rational mind, the logical/analytical part of my brain told me not to be so daft. I began to realise that I had always been over-reliant on this part of my mind, and that to develop I would need to find a balance. The room for growth was in allowing space for my intuitive side - the side that feels and just *knows* without being able prove (and yet somehow doesn't need to prove anything at all). This side is mistrusted and therefore under-used by most of us, but is in fact a pathway to opening up both your world and mind, and countless possibilities.

A critical point at this stage is that having initially recognised these feelings, there is then a need to accept them without further judgement, to take them as being reasonable and normal. In order for this to develop further it is necessary to let this flow uninterrupted within your life, and being sure to avoid the logical analysis that would stop it dead. A rather fitting quote that comes to mind is from the original Star Wars film - "*Use the force, Luke…*".

However corny that might sound, it does somehow seem to capture the essence of it all.

For myself, I am more at the stage of feeling this force rather than using it. This has much to do with nature, and rediscovering your senses. It's about 'un-learning' established assumptions and beliefs, rather than learning anything new, a process of stripping away the layers of civilisation. Take a walk in the woods and breathe, go sit by the brook and be quiet, even get yourself a dog if it helps! See the trees and flowers for the first time - yes, I know how clichéd that sounds, but everything in nature is beautiful when you look at it with your senses in tune with your environment. I mean everything.

Use the force? Well, in time, maybe... You can't train for this, neither can you go looking for it, because you will never find it this way. You can only prepare yourself, open your mind and senses, and be ready to accept this 'feeling'. Then you let things happen in their own time, let things move at their own natural pace.

Certainly this is worth it's weight in gold for finding convenient parking spots, but there are other practical benefits. By being receptive and not trying so hard, I am beginning to find I'm making more of the right decisions. Better still I'm making less of the wrong ones. To be honest I can't always explain why something is the right/wrong thing to do, I just know it to be the case. Later on the reasons will usually reveal themselves, and as long as I have been relaxed, and not consciously looking for an answer, then it has always, **always** been the right choice.

Sounds spooky, but the feeling is one of peace and acceptance. No hocus-pocus, no mumbo-jumbo. This is the 'proper' flow of things.

8. An Equal Footing

An important element in the journey towards becoming a more balanced person, is to gain a better understanding of this life and the world in which we live. We must gain this understanding so that we can start to accept what 'is', and learn how to forgive others. This is essential, as we need to be able to forgive others before we can really understand how to forgive ourselves. These are no more than stepping stones along the path to compassion, however a huge leap is required if we are to find this new level of understanding. To move forwards we need to leave behind the narrow thinking of our past, and accept that everything is much broader than we have previously considered. This acceptance can be a formidable barrier to our development, so to work our way through this we have to go back to the first of those steps, and ask how we might start to gain a better understanding and acceptance of this life and the world around us.

The starting point is to see that we are, ultimately, all equal to one another. That we are all just people. To understand that the boundaries placed by colour, creed, social standing, age, gender, disabilities etc. are completely artificial. Worse, these boundaries are often promoted by people who should know better, and whose blinkered opinions and views are fuelled by nothing more substantial than ignorance or fear. Or often both.

A number of problems immediately spring to mind, including the fact that many of us were brought up with views that were once considered the norm, but are quite rightly no longer acceptable today. There is also the fact we often have little or no experience of some issues, and as a result simply don't know our way around someone else's lifestyle or culture. For example, how do you feel when you see someone in a wheelchair - do you open the door for them? Is this practical assistance or will they be offended by some sort of implication that they can't manage just because they're in a wheelchair? Suppose you meet someone with a disfigured face - where exactly do you look when you speak? How uncomfortable do you feel? Or maybe you meet someone who has difficulties speaking clearly - what do you do, a quick nod and a smile and keep walking...?

Paul Johnson

For myself, I grew up in the 1970s and 80s in a white area of Sheffield. The only kids that weren't white at my primary school were brothers from the one black family in the local area. By the time I moved up to secondary school, an Asian family had also moved in down the street. That was the entire extent of my contact with people from black or ethnic minority backgrounds by the time I left school at sixteen. It wasn't that I had grown up with any particular prejudice, it was just that as I had no experience, these issues hadn't touched my life at all. As a result I had no terms of reference for any of this, no way of differentiating between genuine issues, red herrings, or other people's prejudices. Had I been exposed at that time to particularly strong views for 'this', or against 'that', then I might well have been swayed by those beliefs. It's easy to see how kids are recruited by certain organisations, who make sure they fill the naïve and vulnerable with propaganda for their 'cause'. However, even without such sinister influences, I remained in a state of ignorance until I was exposed to a wide variety of ideas and cultures over the years that followed.

If this was how I grew up, then others must have had similar experiences. I have to say that the easiest choice from this position is to trust what you know, and nothing else. Many people inadvertently make this choice, initially perhaps just through ignorance, which later turns into fear, distrust and intolerance. And so it goes on - building barriers between people and cultures, higher and higher.

Another problem is that although we have all heard of equality, do we actually know what it means? It's a minefield isn't it? The main issues are often assumed to be those of race, gender and physical disabilities, but the list can go on and on - religious beliefs, sexual preferences, political views, age-ism, height-ism, and lots of other 'isms' to boot. Not to mention mental illnesses, learning difficulties, or anything else that might have a less than clear definition. But is this notion of 'equality for all' a god given right or an unreasonable expectation? Is this the sign of a mature and evolved society, or are the weak majority being pushed around by forceful minorities, each with their own blinkered agenda?

Choose Life

An important point that needs to be made at this point, is that Political Correctness (PC) is *not* the same as equality. Not at all. In a perfect world, we know there would be no inequality, and therefore no need for the overt sensitivity that has led to political correctness. Of course in reality this is not the case, so a reaction, and sometimes an over-reaction in the opposite direction was perhaps inevitable. This is often evident at the corporate level, which is where the concept of PC appears to been created. Out of interest, it was recently pointed out (to my amusement) that the term *politically correct* is no longer an 'appropriate phrase'. The correct terminology is apparently now *culturally sensitive* (CS?!). I can only surmise that Political Correctness is no longer politically correct! I'm sure someone is employed in central government somewhere to make this stuff up...

A few years ago, I was surprised to come across the idea that equality does not mean treating everyone equally. I forget exactly where I read this, but I do remember thinking how stupid it sounded. I went on to read the next line (always a good idea), and found it simply stated that equality means that we should treat everyone *fairly*. This was a revelation to me - how simple, how obvious... I mean, surely I could have figured that one out for myself? Treat everyone fairly? No problem. Well, like all theories, it seemed pretty straightforward. And it was. Right up to the point where I tried to match it up with real life.

Do you treat everyone fairly? Strangers on the street, people at work? Training partners in the gym or at the dojo? People that look different, or sound different? What about closer to home, do you treat everyone in your family fairly? Be honest with yourself, do you really...?

One of my kids is profoundly deaf, and her first language is British Sign Language (BSL). We have been signing for a good while now, but thinking back to when we started, it seemed like a pretty strange way to communicate. After a few sessions, our initial reluctance started to give way to a growing enthusiasm, and over the months that followed, our signing gradually became more natural and expressive, and we found this to be a truly beautiful language. For some time we had felt that my daughter was missing out by not having contact with deaf adults and other deaf children - after all despite being part of a loving (hearing) family, she also has a right to be part of the Deaf Community. So, eventually we decided to go to the Deaf Club in Sheffield. We were quite nervous, as the theory of signing in a classroom environment is very different to meeting 'real' deaf people. Also, the nature of BSL is that there are many regional variations on signs, much like we have different regional accents around the country. Except the variations in sign can be totally different, and not recognisable at all. Just the thing to build up your confidence...

So, we arrive at Deaf Club, don't know anyone. Not too many there yet, but people are having a good look at us on the quiet - perhaps they don't get too many new faces in here...? We get in, grab a table and sit down. Got all three kids with us, which gives us a reason to be preoccupied, just while we get used to the situation. Eventually I take a deep breath and walk over to the bar. It's very strange to be in the city I've grown up in, but feeling the same as I might when on holiday abroad. Limited language, and no confidence in using it. Not sure how to order a drink, let alone strike up a conversation. I feel out of place, a stranger in my own backyard.

I get to the bar and manage to order some drinks, a bit of confusion but I just about get by. Not so bad, my confidence starts to lift - hey, this doesn't feel so difficult after all. I'm coming back with the drinks when a woman stops to talk (sign) to me. She asks if me or my family are deaf, I explain, but then she goes into conversation. I can't follow - *sorry, don't understand, say again?* So she signs it again, slowly this time. Still can't see it. Again? Still can't see it. My face is burning now, and my body starting to sweat as panic takes hold.

However, I have a safety net - if all else fails with sign language, you can always fingerspell. That is to spell each letter of a word using your fingers, to explain a sign that someone doesn't know. I can fingerspell, so hey, what can go wrong? Nice lady is being very patient, and decides to fingerspell it for me, save me any more difficulty on my part. Slowly. Oh no, I can't see it - *sorry, again please?* Really sweating now, this woman has just spelled out a five letter word and I couldn't read it. Twice. My confidence is dropping out of my backside now. Please just let me go, please just smile and let me walk on? Oh no, she's trying again…

Later on, and the place has filled up. As a hearing person unfamiliar with Deaf Culture, I could see two quite different social events unfolding in front of me. Firstly we have a large room full of people. Quiet in one sense, because there's no music, and no hum of conversation. At the same time it's actually quite noisy. All these people, rapidly talking with their hands, being able to 'see' other people's conversation from across the room. How strange. I've never heard anything like the noise - screeches, clicks, the intonation of bits of words, shouts and the occasional outburst of laughter. Very strange, and slightly unsettling at first.

Second view of the same situation - by now I've had a couple of pints, relaxed a bit, and had a chance to get used to the scene in front of me. Tried a couple of (brief) signed conversations - not too bad, and my confidence is returning. What does it look like now? A room full of people, all busy, most of them engaged in conversation. Lots of communication going on, right around the room - people drinking and talking, some in serious discussion, others having a real laugh together. Like a pub with a good atmosphere. Ok, so it was different in some ways, but there was a common factor - people. People just going through life, the same as anyone else. Different perhaps on the surface, but just the same underneath. All the usual character types, you know - the good, the bad and the ugly. The kind, the generous, the terminally miserable. The joker in the pack, the selfish, the welcoming and the aloof. All of them in there, just the same as any other group of people. This made me smile, as well as making me think.

We now have a few friends that are deaf. It's funny how things change as you are exposed to new situations and experiences - when I first met one particular couple, the most striking thing about them (as I saw it at the time) was that they were deaf, and that conversation was a struggle for me. Now I think of them first as people, as friends. And as with all good friends, I appreciate their opinions, their sense of humour, and enjoy their company. Oh yes, and by the way they happen to be deaf. Not an issue at all. But when you look at it from this perspective, why would it be? That first visit to Deaf Club got me thinking, mainly about how some people live in very different worlds to that which we usually regard as the 'norm'. Prior to my daughter being born I had never given any thought to deafness, or what impact it had on those affected by hearing loss. It made me think in wider terms, about people who might be less advantaged than myself in some way. If you haven't given this too much thought before, as I hadn't, then try to put yourself in the shoes of someone else, someone facing challenges that are different to yours. For example, try watching the evening news with the sound turned off. Better still watch ten minutes of a video with the sound off, and then rewind and watch it again with the sound back on. See how difficult it can be to understand? And try doing everyday things with your 'wrong' hand, like swapping your knife and fork around at teatime - stick with it for the whole meal if you can. Alternatively try brushing your hair or wiping your backside using the other hand (I strongly advise the use of toilet paper for the latter). Try walking around your own house blindfolded - not as difficult as you might think, but your confidence rapidly disappears when the blindfold goes on. From experience I can say that you're in big trouble if a table or chair isn't in its usual position...

Sounds stupid? Maybe, but this is how life is for some people, only most of us can't imagine. Or rather we haven't tried. So give it a go, see what it's like. Often these things are worth doing just for the experience.

In order to take this whole issue a step further, we need to think of equality as something broader than race, culture, language or disability. It then takes on a different meaning, a different feeling somehow. For example, if we look at this in terms of a martial arts class, how do we tend to treat the beginner, the white belt? Come to think of it, how do we tend to treat a black belt? Remember - it's not about identical treatment, but have we got a basic respect for that person irrespective of the colour of their belt?

Think about it - the white belt in front of you is totally unknown. They may be in fact be a successful businessman or woman, they may have a big and happy family, they might actually have sussed it all out and have much to offer you in terms of understanding how to best live life to the full. They may not of course, but how do you know? In any event, it may not be a question of whether they have achieved those things yet, but if they have the potential to do so (yes, because we all have), where they are currently along that path, and whether you can help them along the way.

That is, of course, ignoring the more obvious question within the martial arts setting, i.e. are they experienced in other arts? I have to confess that I made this mistake many years ago in a Ju-jitsu class, and wasn't really watching the white belt beginner as he threw a punch towards me. After all, I was a brown belt, and was quite experienced (as I thought at the time). Clearly I didn't need to associate any significant threat to this guy. I don't recall what it was that I was thinking about when I should have been concentrating, but suffice to say that I was woken from my daydreaming with a good solid smack in the face!

Staying for a moment in the dojo, how do you treat your instructor? How do you behave towards the visiting 10th Dan Master? This time it is often about their lack of respect for you, an unspoken code that demands your fawning attention or at the very least, a degree of kow-towing. Unfortunately this is often encouraged, if not insisted upon, by many of the instructors themselves. Personally I like to think of meeting this 10th Dan Master (or the company director or whoever) away from their territory, say in the pub, or doing the shopping in the local supermarket. What a great leveller this is - *there's the boss - look, he's buying the same toilet rolls that we get. Hey, he wipes his bum as well! Ha-ha, guess what - we're all just people!!*

Many years ago, I had a 'pub discussion' with a friend, where I explained (with the help of several pints) that within any group of ten people, there would always be about seven or eight 'tossers', leaving only a couple of decent people that I might get along with. Funnily enough I was explaining my own reasons for not discriminating on the grounds of race - in my view there were so many arseholes on this planet, if I started to pick and choose on the grounds of someone's colour as well, then there would hardly be anyone left to talk to. I know, I know... but I was young, and it seemed like a reasonable viewpoint at the time!

The guy I was talking to agreed that colour shouldn't be an issue, however he felt that I had the rest of it back to front. That is to say out of ten people, he expected to find seven or eight decent ones, and perhaps a couple of tossers. With the benefit of the intervening years, I would now be more inclined to agree with the other guy's views. These days I find that most people *do* want to get along with each other - yes, there are always the exceptions, but for the rest it is simply a matter of finding some degree of respect and understanding.

Taking this further, I would probably now give a bit more consideration to the last two individuals, expecting there might well be a decent person hiding beneath the surface. Perhaps they are just socially unskilled, awkward or lacking in confidence. Of course there are never any guarantees, but the likelihood is that there is a decent person in there somewhere. Besides, I have actually been one of those 'tossers' at times in the past, and would certainly have appreciated someone trying to make it easier for me, someone trying to help me out.

My own views on equality have changed a great deal over the years, partly due to getting older, and partly because of my own personal growth and development. Society has also changed significantly since I was a kid - I grew up with the idea that gay men were a disgusting insult to both nature and civilised society, and deserved a good kicking if they got one. To say that now sounds strange, but it was my view at the age of twenty. Fear and ignorance were the main causes (as ever), but it seemed like a reasonable stance at the time. I have to say that I no longer hold such views.

It is strange to leap forward from that to more recent times. For example, only a few years ago on the TV programme Big Brother, the British public voted for an overwhelming victory for Nadia - a Portuguese woman (?) who had undergone a sex change operation. She won the show because the public liked her personality and sense of humour, and could see clearly past the whole gender thing. It is fair to say this could not have happened in the UK ten years earlier, so views do seem to be changing, however slowly.

Choose Life

Recently I was discussing prejudices with a colleague at work, who looked at me rather sceptically when I stated that I don't judge people. Her view was that we all have in-built prejudices of some sort, but we're not very honest about it, even with ourselves. I argued against this at the time, but later thought about it, and realised that she was probably right. Come to think of it, I *do* sometimes make judgements - it could be a particularly obese man coming out of the chip shop *(well there's no need to let yourself get in that state...)*, a group of teenagers wearing hooded tops *(dodgy looking, must be on drugs...)*, or a teenage mum with three young kids *(she must be easy, that one...)*.

You might say that these thoughts are simply cruel or unkind, however there is a further complication. If we consider some of the fundamental lessons in self-protection, such as awareness, avoidance and threat evaluation - these all suggest that it is not only necessary that we make judgements on potential risks, but that such assessments are, in fact, essential. And not just to make a single judgement, but that we should continue to assess and re-assess, as the status of any given situation can change in an instant. Without this ability to continually re-assess, we would be left with 'VICTIM' written right across our foreheads.

So, where exactly does that leave us?

I have to be honest - I'm not aiming at saintliness here. What I do want however, is to treat my fellow man as well as possible, whilst maintaining my own safety, and that of my loved ones. If we were to go back to the obese man, the important things would be what I did, what I actually said, and how I said it. If I'm talking down to this guy, then I really do have a problem. If however, the 'fat man' label dissolves as soon as we start to speak, then I am surely headed in the right direction. A better example might be the group of teenagers, who could potentially be a real threat. I can (and should) avoid any conflict, but I have recognised a potential risk, and will naturally be on a higher state of alert than normal. I may have taken steps to minimise that risk, or to allow a clearer assessment. However, I am also aware that it might turn out to be the kids from next door who I've known for years. I'm conscious that my own children will grow up to be teenagers in time, and may also unintentionally intimidate people. It becomes difficult to see how to balance this against my desire to live and let live.

First things first, there can be no argument with looking after your own safety, as long as this doesn't turn into paranoia. As for finding a balance, the best advice is to not worry too much about the theoretical debates, about whether your fleeting thought of *fat git* or *druggies* makes you a bad person or not. Instead, see how open minded you become as you start to identify the times when you are making unreasonable assumptions, especially when it has no bearing on your safety. *Do* be aware of your environment, and the potential for risks to your well-being, but don't let it stop you from enjoying your life, or treating people with respect. Above all else it is important that you concentrate on treating folk as you would have them treat you. We would all like to be treat fairly throughout our lives, without being targeted for being 'this' or 'that', or conversely for **not** being 'this' or 'that'. It follows that we need to get our own house in order before we have the right to expect this from others, and understand at last that we really can expect to reap exactly what we have sown.

So, when it comes down to it, is equality really a minefield? I don't think so. The bottom line is fairly simple - there are a lot of people in this world, and some of them are different to me. And actually, that's ok.

Keep this in mind and you won't go far wrong.

STEERING THE RAPIDS

Paul Johnson

9. Taking Back Control

Taking back control of a stressful situation can be difficult at the best of times, and harder still if you're caught up in a downward spiral of problems and anxieties. It might seem easy when you read some of the self-help books that are available, with their step-by-step guides and 'revolutionary' techniques. But in practice? Let's be honest here, in practice we all know that it is really difficult. Until recently I would have sighed the heavy sigh of experience, and agreed that putting these things into practise can indeed be pretty tough going. But now I am beginning to realise that this doesn't have to be the case, that your 'truth' can be different if you wish. And best of all, the only thing you will need to achieve this is an open mind...

Following my recent experiences, it would be fair to say that mentally and emotionally I am battered and bruised. Sometimes in charge, at other times like a mass of scars. Sometimes strong, sometimes weak. Even so, I'm still not sure that it has to be all that difficult to take back some degree of control. True, it's always seemed that way, but then again I've always told myself this is the case - that such and such a situation will be tough, stressful, or difficult to deal with. Partly because we've all been conditioned in this way - by other people, their experiences, and also by TV and the rest of the media. The world is full of people who will tell you how hard things are, and of course if you believe them, then you have another negative self-fulfilling prophesy on your hands.

There are also those who proudly wear their stress like a badge, as if proof of what a tough job they have, what a tough life they're having - and, by implication, an indication of just how strong they must be. They are happy to display this badge of office, so that others can recognise their supposed strength and congratulate them on it, or better still, look on with envy. I speak from personal experience - I was one of these people in my last job. For years, come to think of it. Happy to endure this as a symbol of (perceived) seniority, as some sort of proof of importance. Comparing notes and laughing about it with people in the same position, like some sort of exclusive club. Knowing smiles and agreeing that others *just don't understand the pressures*. Well perhaps they don't, but is that a good enough reason to keep on spoiling your own existence? Not to mention the effect on those that really matter, your family and close friends. Let's get one thing straight here - this is about you and those you love, not anyone else. Not the people who don't understand, and certainly not the people who are wearing their stress with pride. There will always be those who carry this right through to the (early) grave, and no doubt they'd be glad of your company along the way. But this is your choice, not theirs. They will make it sound like the sort of exclusive club you must **really** want to be a part of, assuming of course that you *want to be someone*. But in truth this is a nonsense, and the choice will always be yours.

So what now? How do you move this on? Well, for starters, ask yourself why you want to change, make sure you at least understand that much. Forget about past attempts that might have failed, you aren't doomed to automatically repeat your mistakes - this is not Groundhog Day, however much it might feel that way at times. And most importantly, get rid of the negative thoughts. When I catch myself letting negative thoughts or feelings take over, I picture them as smoke in my mind, clouding everything and preventing me from seeing things as they really are. Then in my mind's eye, I feel a gentle breeze blowing through and clearing the smoke. No drama, no excitement, it just quietly drifts away until all is clear.

If you're still unconvinced and perhaps think you can't just change a mood at will, especially when you might be weighed down by some serious baggage, then think for a minute. What about the things that we know have the power to change our moods or emotional states? What about making love? What about alcohol or drugs? Practising meditation or physical exercise? Replaying a bad experience in your mind, or running into an old adversary? What about running into an old friend? Try it now, pick one of these and try hard to visualise it, to imagine this really has just happened. You will be surprised at how you can feel this working - the change in your current mood and the effect on your state of mind. So use the good things, force yourself to replay some of them in your mind. This could be anything from catching up with an old mate, a time when you and your partner got the giggles, or perhaps something funny that your kids said, anything at all. It can alter your mind, your mood - even the rest of your day, so make a habit of it.

Choose Life

This is not dissimilar to using Yin and Yang, as mentioned in a previous chapter, giving different views of the same mountain. A different approach to the same situation, namely that of changing your own perspective to something more positive. Enabling yourself to be feel lighter, happier and be increasingly successful in whatever you are doing.

Back to brass tacks though - how exactly is any of this different from the original well-intentioned advice of *just get on with it* or *pull yourself together?* The main difference is that we have now accepted responsibility for our own actions and thoughts. In doing so, we have seen that stress is not created by the external world around us, and that the biggest single cause of both stress and anxiety is in fact ourselves. To be more precise, it is created by the way we react to the world around us. This immediately becomes exciting...

If we now understand that we can change how we react to external events, then it follows that we can target specific issues that regularly seem to create stress or anxiety, and modify our reactions and attitudes accordingly. Think about it - the goalposts have just moved! No longer is it our aim to stop such situations from occurring, or even to avoid those situations. Instead our aim is to change how we interact with the world. As a result, this has an effect on our own actions and behaviours, our moods and feelings, as well as those of the people around us. In short, this can radically change our overall experience of any given situation.

If I think back to some of the self-help books I have read in recent years, this is probably the part where a book might start to lose me, where I'm not grasping the meaning or context as well as I was in the previous chapters. I have read some excellent books in my time, but when I start to struggle, it can feel like my brain has turned upside down, and is flopping about, gasping for air. This happens to me on a regular basis! When I hit this stage in a book, my usual failing is that I skim through the rest of the chapter, knowing that I'm not taking it in, knowing that I'm missing something of value. The trouble is, I don't want to go back and re-read, do I? Because that would be like admitting I'm not intelligent enough to grasp it at first take, and I'm not admitting that to anyone...

This is stupid I know, but I've done it so many times. The rest of the book then becomes a rush, a competition almost, to race to the end as quickly as possible. But then I never pick up that same book again, and the valuable lessons remain inside, a series of missed opportunities. If this should happen while you are reading this book, then please avoid the temptation to follow my poor example. There is no prize for finishing first and you are not penalised for reading a section more than once...

Going back to the ability to change our experience of a given situation - if we follow this train of thought a little further, we can say that our experiences in life are heavily influenced (at least) by our own attitude and approach. Once you get your head around this stage of thinking, then your perspective suddenly and dramatically shifts. As David R. Hawkins says in his wonderful book *Power vs. Force* - happiness and fulfilment become things that can be found within ourselves, rather than 'out there' someplace.

Read that last line again - *happiness and fulfilment become things that can be found within ourselves, rather than 'out there' someplace.* Wow, this is the sort of stuff that wise men down the centuries have been saying. These are the kind of statements that you can find at the heart of spiritual teachings across the globe, as taught throughout the centuries. What, and it's accessible? To you and me? No need for years of meditation, or living up a mountain as a recluse? You mean we really can access this stuff?

The simple answer is an emphatic YES. Better still, we can access this without leaving the armchair. The liberation that we're talking about is already there, inside your own head. All of the potential is there, waiting for you to tap into it. Right there inside each and every one of us - our birthright, if you like. All you have to do is choose to act. Best of all, there is no such thing as a right or wrong time, in fact you can start right now if you wish. This potential is incredibly powerful - once you open your mind to it you can feel an awakening, a clarity of vision that makes life feel so much lighter. It becomes hard to understand how you've never seen this before.

Astounding, isn't it?

Choose Life

Perhaps even more astounding is the thought that we might not actually need to take control at all. The dawning realisation that this 'need for control' might turn out to be the biggest lie of all, and one that we've all fallen for...

When you look at it, the need to have control over our surroundings actually ends up controlling us. Let's work this through - we start with a perceived need to have control over external events. Our consistent (and inevitable) 'failure' to achieve the desired level of control leads us to feel helpless, powerless within our own lives, not to mention the anxiety that often comes with it. We find ourselves less able to cope with the ups and downs of life, and end up 'fire-fighting', reacting to each new situation or crisis, unable to step back and take a balanced view. Well, perhaps this is unnecessary. Perhaps it is all avoidable.

Why do we need to feel that we are in control of everything? Most of us like to have some routine - yes, this can become dull sometimes, but we generally need a fair amount of routine in order to manage our busy lives. There's nothing wrong with this, as life would be chaotic and stressful without many of these routines, but if we keep going, where does it lead?

Our need for routine and structure seems to be in-built to a large extent. Also, it is likely that much of this is about learnt behaviours and dependencies, impressed upon us by our immediate environment. We've grown up around this, and as a result we don't even see it. But try.

Some of this is doubtless for our own well-being, but hidden within the need for structure and order are a number of less welcome developments. Creativity is stifled. Fear of the unknown creeps in. A dependency starts to grow, an over reliance on the known, on our routines, on the things that are 'safe'. Now, what is the likelihood of you taking a chance? That despite your self-imposed shackles, you will stride out into the unknown to face those challenges, overcome the obstacles in front of you, and become a better and more fulfilled person by doing so?

Not very likely is the answer, because it becomes too difficult, an impossible weight to carry. At times you can see the simplicity of it all. Those who have passed this way before will sometimes show you the true path, and their words cut right through the crap that you've allowed to build up around you. But you're soon dragged back down, to the extent that you lose sight of what those wise men and women were saying. You know what you were going to do, and that only a little while ago it all seemed so easy, but now it's become much too difficult. Now you're wading through treacle once again, and the inspiration has gone.

But what if you didn't have this mountain to climb? What if you could just go directly from point A to point B, without all the internal wrangling and spiralling doubts? What if you could simply take off this millstone that says 'you must have control', and just do it? Imagine - no fuss, no drama, no huge build up. No waiting until your energy levels are up, until you're in the right mood or the conditions are perfect? None of that - imagine if you could just set your sights and go do it.

Well, guess what - you can!

So let's not bother trying to take back control, instead let's use what we have already learnt to apply this idea of 'not needing control'.

In an earlier chapter, I mentioned that I once had an absolute belief that I could overcome whatever might be holding me back, that I would always find a way. It would be true to say that this belief brought me through some real difficult periods, more or less in one piece. But although that might sound like a rock-solid approach, there is an inbuilt flaw, and a serious one at that. An ingrained faith that you will win the fight, often just reinforces the self-made belief that these are difficult times, even that there is a fight to be had.

The other day I unexpectedly bumped into a friend's dad, someone I hadn't seen for quite some time. We chatted for a while, and then at one point he laughed and said *you have to keep on fighting - when you stop fighting, it's all over.* He was part-joking, but it was also a reference to his own attitude. A few days later and I found myself thinking about this. I always had a similar approach, but now I'm starting to see that by always being ready to fight or to do battle, to wave two fingers at the world, the establishment or whoever - this attitude and readiness brings with it an expectation of conflict. In turn this influences your thoughts and actions, and means that you are more likely to bring this conflict about, to make this a part of reality. Despite the fact that your conscious mind would say that this is not a desired outcome.

When I first became aware of this, I made a conscious effort to give up 'being strong'. I let go of the attitude that had got me through my adult life to that point, and became 'nothing'. Not weak, not useless, but without strength, without preset views of what a victory looked like. Or indeed without looking for any sort of victory at all. I just 'was'.

To be honest it was quite alarming at first, like I'd lost a part of me. The part that I knew I could depend on, that I'd always had faith in. Thankfully this feeling soon passed, and I began to find that I was 'observing' myself, as if from outside. Now that I was no longer on autopilot and had stopped using what had almost become preset responses to situations, I could see changes in my own reactions and behaviours - it was amazing to see how many battles just evaporated in front of my eyes. If you don't take part in a battle, then there is no battle. If the outcome, the perceived need for victory is no longer significant, then how exactly can you lose? A victory is there within this 'softer' approach, but as no-victory. You do win, but in a different way, by not buying into this, by neither chasing victory nor fearing defeat. This gives you a totally different perspective, which will then set you free. You are no longer driven or governed by the things that restrict the majority of the population. As a result your thinking becomes freer, and your outlook becomes much broader, both of which then feed into your priorities and actions.

However, there was a drawback. What I seemed to lose was the strict self control, the self-discipline that had been built over years in the gym and the dojo. This had all tied in with being strong and ready to do battle, so when I let go of this strength it was like going into freefall. It took a while to adjust, but then things seemed to be ok, as far as I could tell. It was sometime later before I realised that the self-will and self-discipline that I had relied on for years, had apparently vanished. Along with this softer approach had come weaknesses that I wasn't prepared for. Although I did need to let go of my strength, I began to realise that this new stage was not an end or solution in itself. It was indeed a necessary step, but one that was simply a platform from which to grow.

In truth, there is a need to regain control of some sorts. However, the way to achieve this is by not needing control. To win without winning, to fight without fighting. As frustrating these paradoxes can seem, don't make the mistake of thinking that one thing must be right, therefore the other must be wrong. Instead these are usually different parts of a much bigger picture. It is often the case that we have not yet reached the point where we have the perspective needed to bring this into proper focus, to see the wider picture where such complications and paradoxes no longer exist. But our lack of vision doesn't change what is there to be seen. The wider view of things, the clichéd 'bigger picture' was and always will be there, waiting for our vision to clear. When we realise this, it becomes easier to accept both sides of these apparent paradoxes as being simply the way it looks to us now, at our current level of understanding and consciousness. Then you will not waste any more time dwelling on these matters, nor will you choose a false path by trying so hard to force a 'right' decision.

As you start along this part of your journey, you will begin to find that you *just know*. It's like being weightless - however odd you might find some of this, however it matches (or doesn't) with your current beliefs, just try approaching this with an open mind. Stop making judgment values, stop doubting, stop being rational. Simply stop thinking - try this for a day or two, and see where it takes you. Sure you will be pulled back into rational thinking (old habits really do die hard), but persist, gently put yourself back on track, and enjoy the journey.

Stick with this mindset, even when you start to drop back down into your normal life, and I promise you that nothing will ever seem the same again. And it feels good. Slightly strange at first, but exhilarating, and every bit of it positive. But don't just take my word for it, go and explore this for yourself.

Choose Life

10. Shadow Warriors

The infamous Ninja warriors are surely the stuff of myth and legend. The word itself stirs up a powerful image, however little is widely known about the Ninja. Their recorded history spans some nine centuries, much of which is shrouded in mystery - hardly surprising given that little was known about them at the time, let alone hundreds of years later. One of the most common terms used in connection with the Ninja, is that of *Shadow Warrior*. Usually taken to mean some black-hooded guy, silent and deadly, about to infiltrate the enemy stronghold. Outside the castle walls, blending in with the dark, unseen... Although there is some truth in this, there is also a much deeper meaning to the term 'Shadow Warrior', and one which is very relevant to our journey of personal growth. To examine this, we first need to look at the origins of the Ninja.

For the sake of credibility, I need to say that there are only three genuine Ninja Ryu (with proven lineage) remaining in the world today. The teachings of these schools have been passed down through generations, and bear little resemblance to the Hollywood-type images that we have all seen. The word *Ninja* conjures up a variety of images, often accompanied by a smile or snigger from the average person. And generally a sneer or worse from the average martial arts practitioner.

Despite the all too common misunderstandings, these schools and their teachings essentially consider two things - survival and enlightenment. The forefathers of what eventually became known as the ninja, were not originally concerned with martial strategies or combat techniques at all - these studies were only introduced when it became necessary for the survival of their families. Prior to this, these 'mountain ascetics' were in fact mystics, known for their intuitive understanding of nature, and the ways and intentions of the universe. Exploration of the self, development of the mind and the expansion of perception were key aspects of their studies. Human weaknesses were also studied, both in others, and also looking within. Although this was later changed to incorporate the martial skills necessary for survival, the study of the ways of nature and the universe were to continue, and are indeed still practised today.

From this we can take one meaning of the term 'Shadow Warrior' to be that of facing our own shadows and demons, of searching out our personal weaknesses. And then bringing those weaknesses out into the light, to expose them and start to work with them. The first step, as ever, is that of self-honesty.

To do this, we need to consider our 'dark side' for a moment. Not exactly meaning Darth Vader, but rather that darker side of our minds and personalities. The side that always dwells on the negatives, that eats away at our self-image. The part of our personality that allows the weaknesses of the human condition to grow and fester - guilt, anger, fear, revenge, etc. Although these weaknesses manifest themselves in a myriad of different ways, you can be sure that we all have them.

There is an old Japanese saying that a man has three hearts. The first heart is on display for all to see, and shows only our most public side. The second heart is kept for those who are really close to us, and holds many things that are deeply personal. The third heart, the secret heart, is for ourselves alone, and contains our darker thoughts, forbidden desires and unspoken motives. Not only kept hidden from others, these thoughts are often kept from our own conscious mind. If we are to grow and evolve, then it is vital that the secrets of the third heart are also brought out into the bright light of self-honesty.

Many things may seem to prevent us from taking these steps, but I have to say that it isn't as difficult as you might think. The major obstacle on this path is that of your own pride - the difficulty of starting to admit to yourself that *actually*, you're not quite as good as you might like others to think. Or even as good as you might like to think. If you struggle to face up to your own pride then you will continue to pretend that the shadows aren't there, but however deep we try to bury them, they still exist. There is always a part of us that knows, however deep down, that simply **knows** the truth in these matters. Yes, you can successfully fool yourself for a while, but the honest voice of self awareness will pipe up at some stage. It is up to you whether you stop and listen, or whether you push this down and bury it again. But it comes back up. Again and again.

Choose Life

A concept that is found within most martial philosophies, is that of abandoning the ego. That each of us should let go of all pride and vanity. I took this to heart some time ago, and made a conscious effort to starve my own ego of the attention it craved. Total eradication might ultimately be an impossible task, but after a long and sustained effort, my ego gradually shrunk to the point where it had little control over my thoughts or actions. It felt good to know that when my ego did occasionally pop up and voice an opinion, I would be able to recognise it for what it was. This gave me real freedom, and meant I no longer had to react to people and situations because of my pride, or in defence of my reputation. The clarity this brought was amazing, and it meant I was better placed to make more of the right decisions in my life. All very positive, and very empowering. Surely there can't be a downside to this.

Can there..?

A few years on, and I found myself sharing a couple of beers with a friend called Jeff, a Canadian guy living in England for a while. Jeff is ten years or so younger than me, but my senior in every way in terms of the martial arts. A question comes up during the conversation - do either of us have sufficient confidence and ability to actually use the techniques that we have spent so long practising? Would we be able to perform these techniques in a real life situation, a sudden and unexpected violent encounter? It quickly became apparent that despite years of blood, sweat and tears (literally) in the dojo, we both lacked confidence about the prospect of a live situation. Frustrating.

It was difficult to nail down exactly what was causing this. In my friend's case, we could safely say that he did not lack technical ability. Though fairly young, he possessed an instinctive, effortless movement - I could only train and train in the hope of getting somewhere close to this. In addition to the technical knowledge, he had a keen understanding of awareness and avoidance, and was also well clued-up on of the effects of adrenalin in it's various disguises. So what exactly were we missing? At first we thought it was confidence, but that didn't quite fit. This guy might have been fairly laid back, no arrogance (despite his ability), but he did carry an air of quiet confidence.

No arrogance...? Just a minute, we might have hit on something there. If we look at warriors from any part of the world, from any era, one thing that they all appear to share is some serious self-belief about their own abilities - some pride and ego. Otherwise, how could they have expected to survive a battle, an ambush, a challenge or any other part of an old-fashioned warrior's life?

All right, it is hardly a good thing to be driven by one's ego. Most of us can see that this would not be healthy, after all the perils of being ego-driven are plain for all to see, aren't they? You might have thought so, but unfortunately there are plenty of examples for us to consider, in most walks of life. But if we have no ego (or virtually none), then where does that essential self-belief come from? How can we expect to have the confidence required to get us through the life threatening encounter, or the non-violent conflict that we dread, the scary job interview or whatever else gives us the wobbles?

A trait typical of those interested in self improvement, the 'seekers on the path', is that we often can't see what we have achieved thus far. Always looking ahead, always thinking about the next steps, but rarely feeling any sense of achievement. Never satisfied with our progress to date, or successes along the way. Although we continue to push on with what we believe to be right, we sometimes feel flat, as if there are few rewards for our endeavours. In itself this can cause doubts, and lead us off on to false paths.

Instead then, allow yourself a little time to reflect on your achievements. Allow yourself to say *well done*, give yourself a pat on the back, perhaps even indulge in a moment of pride. This is not only natural, but gives you a lift, a good feeling that can help to provide the energy and motivation for those next steps. In addition, this will also help to start building the all-important self-belief, without which you will struggle to grow and advance, however hard you try.

Without this self-belief you will always be lacking the conviction that is so vital. And in a conflict scenario, there is no room for doubt. All the apparent confidence and ability in the world is virtually worthless when the pressure comes on, unless you have a solid foundation of self-belief. And like it or otherwise, there has to have a degree of ego in there, in order to keep this belief alive. The process of shrinking or starving the ego is absolutely essential if you are to seriously address self improvement, growth and personal enlightenment - but when you *get there*, you then realise this is just another stage. Another stage to be mastered, and then left behind. So having starved the ego down to virtually nothing, the next step is (paradoxically) to start building the ego back up. To a controlled point.

It's a funny old journey - every time you make progress you can think that you've 'made it', but it's never the case. Once you adjust to your new surroundings, your new perspective, then the next steps will become apparent to you. One thing you can be sure of, is that there is always another step, another stage. You can also be sure that it never, ever gets dull!

Back to the traditions of the Shadow Warriors - another concept associated with the Ninja is their idea of 'winning'. Indeed the Bujinkan arts have been accused by others of being dirty, low-down, cheating or somehow unfair. Practitioners of these arts however, fondly refer to them as the 'art of winning'! This is not the notion of winning that we commonly aspire to in the Western world, where a stronger or faster athlete beats a weaker or slower competitor, and usually looks good doing it. Nor is it being perceived as 'better' than those around you, being tougher, stronger, richer, having a bigger house or a better car.

Putting this into the context of a violent confrontation, winning is often thought to mean knocking your attacker unconscious, hitting them so hard that the threat is removed. Well, that's one view. I don't disagree with this, but it is important that we recognise it as only one of the options. Let's suppose the scenario is that you are approached by two guys, one of whom pulls out a knife and shouts at you to give him your money. How do you win? Maybe it is by knocking the guy out, but what if he cuts you before going down? Then again his accomplice might have stuck his own blade into you whilst you were busy dealing with the first guy. Then you end up on the floor, seriously wounded. Not knowing whether it is fatal or just a bleeder, wondering what the kids will say in the morning when Daddy didn't come home. When they realise that Daddy is never coming home. How your partner feels, left to live life alone, and manage bringing up your children without you. So many things left unsaid. So many things said, that never should have been. So much time wasted. Never expected it to end like this, never thought that someone might rob me of forty years of my life. Sod the wallet, someone has stolen my life, and in effect the lives of those close to me. How important do the contents of your wallet seem now? Exactly how does this feel like you have won?

The Ninja ideal of winning is to survive. There is no other agenda, no need to look good doing it, no need to prove anything to anyone, including yourself. Just to survive. From this perspective we can look at the scenario again, and ask again - how do we win? What should we do? How else might we approach this?

Don't think I am about to give you a list of 100% reliable options, never-miss strikes or failsafe moves. There aren't any. Instead look at the main objective again. Having encountered a violent, potentially life threatening situation, I would win by being able to walk through the door of my home a few minutes later, back into the arms of my family, alive.

This really is winning.

And how can we bridge the gap between this confrontation and the sanctuary of home? In truth it is likely to be different each time. In the example used above, the best general advice would be to either hand over your wallet, or if you have the time and space (and a reasonable level of physical fitness), to turn and run. Better still, by living your life with a good awareness of potential risks, you have chosen not to frequent the local 'rough' pub, or not to use that isolated short-cut to the shops. Your choices have ensured that you are not in the wrong place at the wrong time - this is also winning, and is far preferable to facing a violent attacker. However, if a situation should unfold without warning, it might be that you are not able to run - the attack may be on top of you too quickly, or they may want more than your money, perhaps more than you are prepared to give. In this instance you make the choice between curling up and taking it (whatever *it* turns out to be), or you fight. If you choose to fight, then you must do so with every ounce of strength, fear and anger that you have, channel this into a few frenzied seconds, and then take the first escape route that becomes open. Never stay and fight longer than you have to - the longer you stay in the situation, the less likely it is that you will escape.

This chapter has introduced the idea of facing your own shadows and demons, and finding new ways to 'win'. To do this, it is essential that your primary focus at this point is inward-looking - after all, if you are always to be defeated by yourself, then what are the odds for facing external pressures and difficulties?

As tough as this might sound, don't be put off. As with most things, it is simplified by an open mind and a no-nonsense approach. Get this right and you will only need to concentrate on two things. Firstly - self-honesty. Whatever else you do, whatever you tell others, make sure you do not bullshit yourself, as without self-honesty you are lost. If you are prone to kidding yourself, then forget everything else and make this your focus for a few days. Concentrate on it until you are able to look yourself in the mirror, and say out loud, *actually, I do have a problem with (whatever it is).*

Secondly, once you have identified those issues, then you must have the intention to do something about it, and accept that could mean trying more than once.

A lot more than once.

Paul Johnson

11. 'That' Moment

When trying to break out of a cycle of negative behaviour or habits, the most opportune time is when *that moment* arrives. This is the moment when you can sense that the options are being weighed up, that the future is somehow being written. This is the point when the 'new and enlightened you' catches the negative thoughts, escapes the spiral for a few moments, and realises that you could stop. That actually, you are better than this, and don't have to carry on behaving in this way. Usually you will let the moment pass, and go on and have that argument, that drink, that smoke or whatever, knowing that you shouldn't. But don't kid yourself here, this is not spontaneity - this is a choice. A choice that will effectively be made for you if you think for too long without acting. Before you know it, you have missed the moment, and by default will follow what's gone before. This may well be down to habits and well established routines, ingrained behaviours or even history repeating itself. But even so, you know that moment existed. Even if you didn't act, you knew the moment was there, and that is all the potential you need to make changes in your life.

When I arrived at that moment a while ago, I took a deep breath and told myself that none of the thoughts in my head were real. I told myself that none of the pressures existed, and there was no predetermined outcome, because all of this existed only inside my head. And nowhere else. A surreal moment followed where it all just fell away, melted away into nothing, and I could **really** see. Actually I can do anything. Anything at all. All of the limitations are either ones I have placed there myself, or are just my perceptions of what other people *might* think. It's false, all of it. When you strip things right down, there really are no limits. At this moment I had more clarity than at any other point in my life, and the funniest thing is that it was all so easy. All of it, so easy, so simple that it seemed ridiculous to think I have let these things affect my life for so long. At that moment it was **so easy** that it was inconceivable that these things could ever cloud my judgement or get in the way again.

But back on planet Earth, back into the reality of day-to-day life - is it really that easy? An honest answer would be that when you keep your mind clear and in the present, then yes, it is easy. Ridiculously easy. But it does need working at, as the thoughts, the internal arguments and downwards spirals *will* keep coming. This is just human nature. What you have to remember is that every time you get a grip, you become stronger. Every success, large or small, will build your strength, and in doing so will make the next time easier to handle.

And when you do get bogged down in the negative stuff? Don't worry, you've won just by realising, and that gives you the opportunity to think and act differently. And the best bit is that you don't ever need to beat yourself up when it goes wrong, because this is more time wasted, more energy-sapping arguments that exist only inside your head.

STOP.

That's all, just stop. Stop thinking, then say out loud - *well done, I've done good there. It was hard at first, but I got control of that one. I actually did alright there...*

A few weeks on, and I'm able to reflect on this. What I'm starting to find is that although this 'moment' does keep appearing, it's more obvious now, and it stays for a while. Instead of just being a fleeting moment that disappears if I hesitate, it stays for longer, almost as if someone hits the pause button for a few minutes. Life does carry on around me, but the feeling of the future being written, of decisions being made - that part goes on hold.

Result? Once again I have more time to make the right decision, to take the positive route. And of course because it's becoming easier, I find myself taking this route more and more often. Although this seemed weird at first, it has gradually become a normal part of my life. The whole process is more relaxed. In a way it is almost building itself - positive leads to positive leads to positive. The complete opposite of the vicious circles that have held me back for years.

Sometimes I wonder exactly where all of this is going, where it's taking me. And then I stop. I remember where I was a few short months ago, and realise that it's enough just to be free. Maybe it doesn't matter too much where I'm going. Things feel fantastic now, so why spoil things by worrying too much about the future? I'm not sure when I last felt any serious anxieties, although now that I think about it, those feelings seem to have stopped coming. Same with the stress - not such a dramatic change, as some of it still needs to be 'dealt with' at times, but it is certainly nowhere near the debilitating levels that I was living with a sort time ago. Put into that perspective, it feels better and better to be alive. And as for where this is going, for now I am happy to sit back and enjoy the ride. A kind of magical mystery tour, I guess. Sometimes it's like being a kid again, living in a wonderful world, where everything is exciting and free.

It occurred to me recently that there are other, less obvious times that might also be one of 'those moments'. These are much less dramatic, but seem to crop up more often. The times when you know you should speak, should interrupt or take the initiative, but generally don't. Sometimes you bite your lip and let the moment pass, and then beat yourself up afterwards. Sometimes this will go around and around and around in your head for the rest of the day, because you are disappointed, embarrassed or even angry with yourself for not having dealt with things better. Funnily enough, it usually follows that you're never quite sure **why** you didn't deal with it better. These incidents can be anything from small-scale and petty right through to the major life-changing variety. Irrespective of the scale, the most common reason for allowing these moments to pass us by is a lack of courage. Short of bottle. Lacking moral fibre. After some reflection on my own experiences and shortcomings, I began to look for examples of real courage. I wanted to find inspiration and motivation, to see real-life examples that I could learn from. I am not talking about a fearless mountain climber here, or a big, brave deep-sea diver, but instead examples of true courage in an *ordinary* life setting. After all, it's one thing to be brave at a time you have planned and prepared for, but quite different when the twists and turns of life catch you unprepared, leaving you frozen like a rabbit in the headlights.

The biggest examples that I found turned out to have one thing in common - they all involved children. For example, the quiet courage shown by the six year old having to sleep with an oxygen mask strapped to his face. Not panicking when he vomited in his sleep at 3am, the oxygen mask filling up with sick because his dad wasn't quick enough. Not panicking when his air supply was cut off, and hot vomit was running out around his head, through his hair and clothes. Somehow keeping his cool when most adults would have freaked out.

Then there's the three year old who was in hospital for major surgery, including drilling into her back of the skull. She was up and about that same day, wobbling up and down the ward, wanting to play with (and look after) the 'poorly children'. And also their brothers and sisters who wait at home, upset and drawn in, but never understanding properly, especially the younger ones. Left managing their own emotional turmoil, because mum and dad might have been trying their best, but were in crisis themselves and unable cope with so many conflicting needs. However hard they might have tried. Very young kids struggling, growing up too quick, taking on board confusion and upset, and just having to accept it. All the attention might have been on the older brother/sister in the hospital, but the ripples affect so many others. This is a different kind of courage.

Don't think this is a reference to some dodgy Yuletide telly programme, with Rolf or Cilla visiting poorly kids in hospital on Christmas Day - the sort of thing that gets you in the heart and throat, but disappears when you change channels for something less disturbing. This is closer to home. Much closer.

I am the dad that wasn't quick enough, that was stroking the sick-covered hair, trying to sound cool and calm whilst panicking like hell inside. I am the dad that looked on with pride and wonder as my bandaged daughter wobbled off down the ward to look after the 'poorly' kids. And I am the dad that wondered (and still do) at the way my youngest has handled all of this and more in her little life, and guiltily hope that it has no lasting effect on her. I know for sure that I wasn't as brave as my kids were at these moments, all three of them were out of this world - each of them showing bravery and strength beyond their years. This is real courage.

But now I have to stand back and ask why?

Choose Life

Why is it that young kids can demonstrate such levels of bravery and courage in terrible situations, but we adults are often left struggling? One of the main reasons seems to be that our children generally have faith that the adults are largely in control of the situation. Perhaps less so as they get older, but this is very much the case for younger children. My own kids have some degree of faith, especially in a crisis situation - so if I tell them it is going to be ok, then it probably is. If I say things are alright and there's no need to panic, then as long as I sound like I **really** mean it, then they will accept this at face value. Children are usually able to do this because there is someone else involved, someone that they trust. The bottom line of course is that this isn't their responsibility. As they see it, the buck stops with someone else. It is much easier to have the necessary courage when you have this level of trust, and the feeling that someone else is in control, taking charge of things. This is not meant to take anything away from the kids themselves - I think they are absolute stars, however it is quite enlightening to understand how this works.

As adults, we usually hold the responsibility ourselves. The buck does stop with us, and we often have little faith that things will work out. Many of us are worn down and jaded by life's let-downs and disappointments, so we 'protect' ourselves by expecting a negative outcome. After all, if you don't expect too much, then you can't be disappointed when things don't work out, right...? As adults, there are very few who have anyone feeding us with positive messages, building our strength and resilience, and telling us that everything is going to be alright. Sometimes it would be nice.

So, if this is where were are - lacking in faith, and short of courage as a result - then where do we go from here? How do we build on these shaky foundations? A colleague at work has a saying pinned up in front of her desk:

> *Be brave. If you don't feel brave, pretend.*
> *No-one else can tell the difference.*

This is an exceptionally practical piece of advice. It helps bridge the gap between knowing that the moment is there, and taking that first step. Probably the only time I would advocate hiding from the truth of a situation. We need to be clear that this 'hiding' is not about fooling other people, but is instead something that we can use to build our own capabilities. If you appear to know what you are doing, to be entirely capable, then others are more likely to believe in you. As a result they will react more positively, enabling you to make more of a success of your chosen endeavour. Also, once you have established this 'alleged' confidence, then you place an unspoken expectation that your actions will live up to this. Not only for others, but also for yourself, especially for yourself. The expectation that your actions will lead to the positive outcomes that you are portraying in your 'role play', in turn propels you beyond the limits of your comfort zone. This is a major step towards living up to our potential, that which is within each one of us whether we can see it or not, whether we choose to acknowledge it or not. This wonderful potential resides within us all, just waiting to be uncovered.

One word of warning though - it is sensible to employ a little caution, as there is a risk of over-committing, of biting off more than you can chew. When we do this, it often leads to failure, with the inevitable come-backs of *told you so*, and *who do you think you are?* At the same time, you must not let this hold you back too much - that would be fear, disguising itself as the sensible voice of caution. There is a balance that must be struck here, so you must be sure to find the middle ground.

My first experience of 'pretending' in this way came when I made the step up from 'worker' to 'supervisor' - I took over my boss' job when he moved on, so this was a step taken within the same team. On one hand it was great that I already had a good relationship with most of the team, but on the other hand, they all knew that I had no experience as a manager. In addition, one or two of these guys had gone for the same job, only to be beaten to the post. There might not have been any outward sign of hostility or resentment, but I knew it was there, under the surface.

In the first place, I tried to do a lot of listening, and consciously avoided the temptation to immediately stamp my own impression on things. I set out to understand the strengths in what was already in place, as well as the more obvious weaknesses, but in those first few months I was winging it, and everyone knew it. Granted, for the most part they were quite supportive, but they all knew that I was making it up as I went along. As the weeks passed, I realised that the guys were sometimes uncomfortable, even embarrassed for me when I found myself left high and dry without a clue. Worse still if I admitted it, as I no longer had the excuse of *hey, I'm just a worker, the same as you guys*. What I hadn't twigged immediately was that they wanted me to act according to my role.

It doesn't matter what the specifics are - it could be a manager, a teacher, a mechanic or a nurse. A mother, a plumber, a dentist or a policeman. Think about it - don't you have a predefined role in mind for each of these? What I realised was that people wanted me to play the part, to behave like a real manager, even though they knew otherwise. And even though they knew that I knew that they knew, if you see what I mean. Despite all of this, in order to be comfortable, the guys in the team wanted me to behave in a manner that they associated with the manager's role.

When I realised this, I decided to role-play, to pretend, to guess - based on past experiences with my own managers, both good and bad. Work out what to do, how to act, and especially how to speak to the people around me. In effect those people, especially their feelings and opinions, had become my working material. These were the things I would have to work with, mould and flow with in order to achieve any decent results - quite a change of perspective from my previous life as a 'worker'. Of course, I wouldn't be able to do this if people weren't comfortable, and for that to happen they needed me to act out the role of a 'proper' manager, to meet their need for a familiar routine. Yes, there was room for individual style, but the basics needed to be covered - change too much too quickly, and people become uncomfortable.

So we started to play along. And it felt strange. They were well aware that I didn't know what I was doing, but happy for us to carry on with the pretence, as it created a more comfortable situation for everyone. The basic requirement was to avoid playing the role of the well-intentioned but disastrous new manager *(hey, everyone, I really don't know what I'm doing)*, to act more confidently in unknown situations, and to appear both relaxed and decisive whilst secretly trying not to panic. I wasn't aware at the time, but this was actually building me up, day by day, week by week. As I gained more positive experiences, my confidence grew, which in turn led to more positive outcomes, then more growing confidence, and so on - you get the picture, this began to feed itself, to take on a life of it's own.

After a while, you either reach a point where you can't keep up the pretence anymore - usually because you have chosen to act in a way that is too far removed from your own personality to be sustainable - or the line between pretence and reality starts to blur. This can be a little strange, as you are not aware of the change until some time later. You eventually realise that you have played the role of (let's say) a more confident and decisive person for so long, that it has changed you as a person. Permanently. Instead of continuing to act out this role endlessly, you have actually become a more confident and decisive person. Although at times you might feel the 'new you' starting to disappear, this is fine, because you then automatically pick up the role-play and start consciously acting again. Although as time passes, you will find this happens less and less.

This is a very effective way to make positive changes - so much of our behaviour is ingrained, and the result of being a certain way or reacting in a particular manner for so many years, that we have to actively re-train our subconscious mind. But it can be done. And best of all, it isn't all that hard to do - all it takes is persistence. And a sense of humour.

When you do find yourself in what might seem to be a difficult situation, it often helps to think in the third person - as if someone other than yourself is dealing with things. In the situation above for example, you could think of this in terms of summoning up a more confident 'you', a bold decisive character who takes responsibility in their stride, who makes strong decisions without fear, without crumbling under the perceived pressure. This is not a million miles away from the approach of some Buddhist traditions, which study different aspects of human nature in isolation from the whole, with a focus on both the positive and negative sides of an emotion or character trait. Meditative study enables a deeper understanding of all aspects of a particular attribute, how it affects our lives, and how any apparent negatives might sometimes be positive, and vice versa. In addition, they will 'call up' a character (not a god) that epitomises the positive aspects of a given area of study.

For example, in Mikkyo (The Japanese Diamond and Lotus Tradition) the character named Kongosatta has the ability to see clearly, to take a detached scientific view of a situation. Fudo Myo-oh characterises righteousness, and is tough, immoveable, resolute. Another example would be Kokuzo, who has the ability to see beyond face value, beyond the obvious, and grasp the essential essence of a situation. Forget about the odd-sounding names and think for a moment about what these characters represent. Have you ever felt that you could do with some help when you are feeling weak, when you start to wobble? Would you have liked to be able to summon up someone solid, something to help steel yourself when you started to waver? It would have helped me at many times in the past. These characters are actually no more than a reflection of our own unexplored capabilities, although it is often useful to see them as something external that we can 'call up' when needed.

Alternatively, if that should feel uncomfortable for you, then you might try a different approach - one that helps many people is to find a role-model. Ideally this would be someone who has been through some difficulties in their life, taken a few hard knocks, but is still standing and living life to the full. This person could be anyone, but it must be someone that you respect, that has a positive influence on you. It could be someone you already know - a friend, teacher, family member or work colleague. Equally it could be someone that you respect and admire from a distance - a writer, martial arts instructor, a rock climber, painter or whatever.

Importantly, once you have found the right person to model your behaviour upon, you must allow them to remain human. That is to say don't make the mistake of expecting perfection from them, don't build them up in your imagination to be some god-like figure that can do no wrong. This would surely lead to disappointment. When you have built someone up this way, it almost feels like a betrayal to find out that they are just a person after all, that they still have their failings. So pick the right influences, but allow them to remain imperfect - that way a good role model can help you, whether directly or indirectly. They can guide you to make the right choices and help to build your inner strength and beliefs, without you becoming too attached (or borderline obsessive!). Use their positive influence to help shape what you already have, and help you to grow into yourself, rather than trying to become a carbon copy of your 'hero'. Finding a positive role model is very empowering, as it gives you somewhere to check-in when things get tough - a reference point and a much needed source of inspiration.

However potent these different approaches can be, it is important that we also retain our perspective, and keep sight of the fact that this drive for personal improvement and development is continuous. It is not about arriving at some glorious destination, in truth there isn't one. There never was. The rewards will come along in their own time, in tune with the proper flow of things - this is something you can count on, and therefore allow your focus to be on each step of the way ahead, rather than on the expectation of rewards. Building up hopes of absolute perfection will only lead to disappointment and misery, instead the right way is one of small steps, of continually moving forwards. This includes the acceptance of occasional failures, big or small, but never being distracted long enough to stray off the path. Never grinding to a halt, always moving - always stepping forward, whatever the speed.

I have to say that cliché or otherwise, life really is about the journey. Satisfaction in life truly comes from our experiences along the way.

12. Achilles' Heel

This talk of facing one's own shadows, recognising 'that moment' and avoiding the cop-out is all good and well, but there is a danger that it could come across as smug-sounding advice. The sort of stuff I might have read in the past and found myself unable to relate to the day-to-day realities of my life. Things often seem far from straightforward when you take the step from theory to real life, especially considering that we all have our own context for this - that of our individual weaknesses and vulnerabilities.

For many years, my own Achilles' heel has been alcohol. Not particularly unusual, as this is a very socially acceptable drug, and is widely used for a variety of reasons. However it is surprising just how much you can drink without anyone being unduly concerned. My own struggles around this, and the fact that we find such problems so difficult to discuss, serve to make this chapter deeply personal.

Picture the scene. It's Sunday lunchtime on the motorway, heavy traffic moving slowly through the road works. We're doing perhaps 20mph, and my head is out of the passenger side window, vomiting. Repeatedly. Can't pull over as the hard shoulder is coned off, and an extra lane is about to join from our left. Nowhere to hide. We're going slow enough that the vomit doesn't all blow back in my face, but still fast enough that it goes all over the exterior of the car. The heavy traffic means there are plenty of people to watch my performance, especially with the extra lane about to join from my side. I decide not to make eye contact with my audience, and keep on looking down at the tarmac, pretending that I'm not aware of them. Not nice, not at all. I'm really not sure that last night was worth this humiliation.

Yep, the result of overdoing it with the beer. I'd had a couple of lagers in the house, then got a phone call out of the blue from some friends, and shot off to meet them in the pub. Catching up, drinking, talking, drinking. Time goes on hold, tomorrow doesn't exist, and you somehow get younger and younger as the night goes on. Binge drinking - a fine old British tradition.

Alcohol has always had a special place in my life. I've never been an alcoholic, but have always managed to drink more than is either wise or healthy. *A special place in my life?* Now that is starting to sound scary. It's true though. In fact alcohol has served me well through many a difficult period, held me together, got me through a few hard times. Hey, you could almost say that it is my special friend... *cut to mental images of Homer Simpson cuddling a crate of Duff beer.* Hmm, I'm not entirely sure this is showing me in my best light...

To understand my relationship with alcohol, you have to go back to 1986. Sixteen years old, we're all outside the pub, working up the courage to go in and order a pint. Looking back, we were just kids. A few quid in our pockets because we were all working, determined to be 'grown ups', and determined to have a good time doing so. A good time that could only be achieved in one way - the traditional British way of drinking as much beer as possible, and as quickly as possible, before the (then) short opening hours see the bell ringing for last orders. God forbid that should happen before you are completely bladdered - if you finish the night without being totally wrecked, then you simply haven't had a good time.

It wasn't just us teenagers starting out, the pubs were full of 'proper' grown-ups doing exactly the same on a Friday and Saturday night - a bit of escapism. Easing away the pressures of the week, and trying to alleviate some of the pain and boredom. And so it went on, for years and years. Not only was this an acceptable way to drink, it was the only way for most of us. Why? Because (as we all know), the single purpose of drinking is to get hammered. Absolutely annihilated. Otherwise, you haven't had enough. Straightforward enough for me, and over the years that followed, I certainly put the hours of practice in.

Although the U.K. licensing laws have since been relaxed, this type of binge drinking remains the norm for many people. Like it or not, this is a part of British culture, and one that will remain for many years to come. Now I might be older and wiser, but the years seem to drop off when I approach a bar. By the time I get served, I feel like I'm eighteen again, all revved up and raring to go, ready to push my limits. Pathetic? Maybe, but I guess this is symptomatic of spending my late teens through to late twenties drinking in this manner.

There are (inevitably) many entertaining stories that come to mind - a wide variety of outrageous drunken exploits to be recalled. It goes with the territory. Despite the humour value, however, I have decided not to tell all. It's better that way, as I can hang on to what little remains of my dignity. Besides, you might not really want to know about the embarrassing memory blanks, my personal vendetta against Ladas, or how a giant turd came to be sitting in my bath one morning...

Jump forward in time to 1998 - a year after we had moved into a new area. We had never quite got into the pub scene after the move, largely because my wife was pregnant, and it just didn't seem right. So we had finally broken the routine, and the cycle of weekend pub binges came to an unexpected end. Clearly the problem was solved.

If only that had been the case.

It is a strange thing for someone who has always liked a drink to find themselves without either a pub or a willing drinking partner. The situation did however help me to realise that the whole weekend drinking thing had become dull and jaded over the years. That I wasn't enjoying it as much as I used to, and had just been going through the motions. We had been in our new home for just over a year, and although we hadn't found the rhythm of the local pub-life, we had just been through one of the biggest life changing experiences that it is possible to have. Our first child. Exhilarating, exciting, astounding. Scary too. A great deal of positives, to say the least, but so very, very tiring. Any remaining doubt about the pub scene was finally laid to rest by the exhaustion. We suddenly found ourselves so bone-achingly tired that neither of us had the motivation to go out. To be honest we really couldn't be bothered to make the arrangements, let alone the effort to actually get ourselves ready. It had no meaning at that point. Our new life was good, wonderful in many ways, but the days and weeks just melted together in a bleary-eyed haze. Notions of going drinking and socialising seemed as alien as a little green man in a spaceship.

So - no more alcohol then? For a short while it seemed to be the case, but then I discovered the joys of drinking at home. And it's not as if I had to drink a lot, just two or three would do, no harm in that. *Wow - look at the prices up the off-license, it's so cheap compared with the pub, they're almost giving it away. Blimey, might as well get a few down me at this price, eh? The more you drink, the more you save.* Well, it kind of seemed that way at the time.

Sometimes I drank a fair bit, sometimes just a couple, and often nothing at all. After all I had to get up for work in the week, so my drinking was mainly restricted to the weekends. Just common sense really, and for a while the notion of drinking in the house seemed to be a reasonable adjustment from our old life to the new. But then things got more complicated as other issues started to appear. Life with one, then two, then three young children is tough. Issues appear around health - eczema and asthma, serious food allergies, physical disabilities and hearing impairment, all on top of having a very young family with insufficient support around us. Life is hard, more so than I could ever have imagined. No regrets, not ever - having kids is the finest and most rewarding thing that we have ever done, and gave us a real purpose for life. Whatever the clichés, when it happens for you (and when this is what you want), having kids is the most rewarding and fulfilling thing that can happen to you. It can also be the hardest.

Around the same time, lots of pressures at work are adding to the fun, and as a result I sometimes feel like I deserve a little reward by the end of the day. Nothing heavy, but just a little something to say well done, got through another tough day in one piece. To someone else, this might have been a cream cake and a weight problem, or an eating disorder. But for me, this inevitably took the form of a couple of beers. The problem here is that you get used to having a drink in the evening. At first it's just sometimes in the week, then it becomes more days than not. Later on and it's almost every night, later still and you realise that you're kidding yourself with the 'almost'. Of course there is the occasional worry that you might be overdoing it a little, but that's easy sorted - you can prove to yourself there is no problem by going without for a night or two, and then happy once more, you can have a drink again the next night. Or two. And so it continues.

Choose Life

It's difficult to remain in a state of denial for long, especially when you are taking a long, hard look at your own shadows and weaknesses. In the cold light of one hung-over morning, I found that I could finally admit to myself that I have a problem with alcohol. A real problem. Can't be a physical addiction though, because I've already proved that I can abstain for a few weeks. Also, no matter how much I've actually been drinking, it has always been exclusively in the evening. I've never liked daytime drinking - a good job really or I might well have been a full-blown alcoholic. The biggest difficulty now is to understand exactly what the problem is.

The way I use alcohol to self-medicate was once described as using an 'emotional anaesthetic'. It took me a while to figure that one out, but it really doesn't capture the nature of my drinking at all. Yes, I am drinking for effect, self-medicating to cope with the pressures of a busy stressful life. But what it actually does is to suppress the feelings of stress, of not being able to cope, and allow me to see (and feel) what is really beneath this difficult surface layer. This actually creates another problem, as I quite like what's underneath, quite like this perspective. Unfortunately, it seems I can only access this by poisoning myself every night. Can't be right.

Cutting down is the usual advice, however it just doesn't work for me. I know that I drink too much, too often, and for the wrong reasons. Reducing my intake makes perfect sense, but I've been around this loop too many times before and ultimately it hasn't made a difference. Recently I tried this again, decided to cut out the drink for a few days. I made this decision made on a Sunday afternoon - no more beer until Friday night. I've managed to do it before, so it shouldn't be too hard.

Fast forward to that evening and where am I? In the off-license as usual. Only this time it's not for the usual few cans of lager or a bottle of red - this time I've bought a big box of wine. The equivalent of four normal bottles. You know the stuff - cardboard box, little plastic tap on the side, keep going by the glass. No idea how much you've had until it's empty a few days later. Even then, no longer certain how much you had. Or when. So not only have I abandoned my decision to stop for a few days, I have positively waved two fingers at it by going **way** over the top. I might know that it isn't the right thing to do, but somehow I can't seem to stop myself.

The next day I start thinking about this - why does it have to be this way, what it is that drives me to self-destruct? There's also this tendency of mine to fight my way through life, to create unnecessary battles, and I'm wondering now if it just might apply to this situation. Maybe this is why I always return to drinking. Maybe this is why I always revert back to having a bit too much, a bit too often. This is not really about alcohol, that's just how it is coming out, how the problem is presenting itself. This is about an internal battle. This is about me fighting myself. Exactly the type of internal battle that I talked about earlier - self-created and self-destructive.

But despite all of this self-learning, this new found awareness, I still can't control my drinking. This is no way to live - it simply doesn't make sense. You can see the direct parallels with people who get caught up in a cycle of endless dieting, but never quite manage to change their lifestyles, and as a result never succeed in the long term. Just the same issues under the surface here. But what do you do? I thought I had been growing in my understanding, thought I had made a few major breakthroughs along the way - but now it feels like I have achieved nothing. I am still being driven by the most basic of impulses, and this lack of control is impacting on my health, my life, and the well-being and harmony of those around me. It's low level stuff really, hardly the sort of thing that should stop me in my tracks on this supposed path to a better life.

Self-development - who am I kidding? It takes more than reading a couple of interesting books to reach a state of enlightenment. You need to do something positive with that learning, make a difference in your life. And if you can't get a grip on the most basic of impulses, desires, or addictions, where does that leave you? All the knowledge in the world is of little use if you can't apply it.

So now I'm rock bottom, and I'm not sure how I can get back up this time. My push along the self development/personal growth route has been a real motivator, helped get me back up and moving again. But now it feels like I've hit a wall. A real solid wall, you know the sort - can't go under it, can't go around it, can't go over it. It is so much bigger than I am, so very much bigger, and here I am with no answers. On the floor again after all this time. After all those dreams of a better life, of changing myself, of changing the world around me.

And here I am.

Fucked.

Paul Johnson

Choose Life

SPREADING WINGS

Paul Johnson

13. The Martial Arts

What do the martial arts mean to Joe Public? Kung-fu kicks and Bruce Lee moves, quick-fire punching complete with sound effects. High spinning kicks and amazing leaping attacks, fancy throws and heavy landings. Big-Arnie super strength and smart one liners, Jackie Chan humour and impossible odds. Supreme self defence - knocking out opponents with single strikes and unlikely kicks. Having the ultimate spirit, grit and determination, taking massive hits and knockout blows then getting back up with no more than a grunt, as if superhuman. The awesome black belt - able to take out a whole platoon of marines with one hand behind his back, yet without causing serious injury. Not to mention the legendary Death Touch - taught to very few, but able to cause death within hours by nothing more than a slight touch.

And what of the thousands that train each week, in a wide variety of styles and environments - what do the martial arts mean to them? Confidence, self awareness, self improvement. Learning to hit, learning to move, learning how not to be hit. Self defence, fitness, technical knowledge. The sheer pleasure of the training. History and tradition, the arts of war. Fighting. Fighting without fighting. The mental challenge, overcoming difficulties, facing fears. Friendships, being part of something, belonging. Bonding and growing, individually and as a group. The black belt - often seen as the goal by those yet to attain it, usually seen as the beginning by those who already have. Personal development, spiritual enlightenment, becoming a better person. Finding the flow of the universe, understanding one's role in this world, knowing how to influence those around you for the better.

Hard to imagine a greater gulf between public image and reality, isn't it...?

For myself, I found the martial arts almost by accident. I quit smoking in the early nineties, and soon started to look for some sort of sports activity to improve my fitness. Having talked on the phone to a Ju-Jitsu guy in Chesterfield, my curiosity was tweaked enough to make a visit worthwhile. I had no idea what to expect, absolutely none, but was enthralled by what I saw. A love affair with the art immediately followed, and I was to stay for some five years or so.

Prior to this I had grown up with a strange mixture of overt confidence in known situations, combined with fear and an inability to think (or sometimes to even speak) in unknown/uncertain situations. I was particularly uncomfortable and timid with people that I didn't know - a lack of confidence, uncertain self image and inadequate social skills conspired to make life difficult. Those that knew me well thought I was all upfront and confident, without seeing that this was only one side of me.

No-one seemed to ever realise how difficult I found unknown situations, or how hard it could be to speak to people - especially with social chit-chat. I seemed to be the only person incapable of dealing with such ordinary day-to-day conversations. The more socially skilled might find it difficult to understand this polarised behaviour, of being apparently outgoing and confident, but then unable to make small talk about the weather because of my awkwardness. It could be hard enough with blokes, but even more difficult with women. Not comfortable, and definitely not good for you.

Over the years that followed, my time with the Ju-Jitsu club really seemed to help. My confidence grew, and I started to find it easier to talk to people. I threw off the shackles of a poorly paid job, went out into a new and growing industry, and found ways of pushing my boundaries on all sides. This was a very exciting time for me. What also developed, although I'm not sure I was aware at the time, was some degree of self-belief. During this period I trained hard and consistently, accepted pain and discomfort as being the price of knowledge, and absorbed a great deal from the instructors. As my technique developed, my confidence also grew, and with it, the belief that I would be able to use these skills should I ever need to defend myself. In turn, this unquestioning belief enabled me to learn and progress well within my chosen system, and so it went on. However this was not to last.

After about four years or so, I started to question the practical value of what I had learnt. Yes I was fairly confident in my ability in a

Choose Life

dojo setting, but what about in the street? What if I was attacked? What if it was by someone who had done some boxing, or an experienced street fighter? The Big Question - the one that had lingered unwelcome in the back of my mind for so long - finally forced it's way out. Exactly what is this black belt worth in terms of **real** self defence?

My instructors at the club were good people, and technically very able, but felt they had to be seen to have all the answers. This lack of honesty on their part was then fuelled by the increasing influence of those who were (at the time) starting to challenge the traditional arts, and question the validity of their claims to teach effective self-defence. So how would I really fare against a boxer? What is this black belt actually worth? The answers that came out in the cold light of honesty were to leave no room for excuses. The art I had spent years studying, in the final analysis, turned out to be built on unstable foundations. Foundations which would not have stood up in the face of real violence.

My self-belief was in pieces, my confidence shattered. *What should I do, just carry on, and hope this goes away? How can the other students and teachers keep their eyes and minds closed to this? Don't tell me they've never wondered. The (alleged) applications that we are being taught don't actually stand up under pressure - surely this must concern them? And what now - do I just walk away? Will having nothing be better than having this?* There were no easy answers, but after long months of anguish and internal wrangling, I eventually decided that I had no option other than to walk away from the art I loved. I felt crushed and betrayed. Absolutely devastated.

This was the start of two years mourning. I made occasional disappointing visits to check out various clubs, ranging from Kick Boxing to Hapkido, Free-style Karate to Aiki-jutsu, but never anything that felt real. Not a day passed when I didn't feel upset at having lost the art I loved. Other wonderful things came into my life during this period, in particular my growing family, and needless to say this did much to distract me from the martial arts, and brought great joy into my life (which continues to this day). But the feelings of loss, betrayal and grief were always there beneath the surface.

Paul Johnson

Finally I stumbled across a poster advertising a martial art - not one I'd heard of before, but one that claimed to be about real combat, with no sports application whatsoever. It sounded worth a visit, and what followed was another love affair, this time with Bujinkan Ninpo Tai-jutsu - a Japanese combat art, incorporating nine separate traditions (ryu) under one Grandmaster. This included ancient Samurai ryu, and Ninja ryu, along with a wide variety of weapons. This unique combination of martial traditions also had a genuine focus on survival in the widest sense. In addition, the spiritual aspects of the art were openly discussed - rather different from my previous experiences. Personal enlightenment and spiritual development were considered an integral part of the journey. Immersion in these arts provided a path towards becoming a complete and enlightened human being, not just a master of martial technique. The ultimate goal is one of true personal power, described as *attaining the mind and eyes of God*.

On the physical plane, the training had much to do with unlearning old ways, and was big on spontaneity. Learning to relax, to move, and to change techniques mid-flow when needed. A real change from the physically strong techniques I had previously learnt. This was an art that would take your opponent to a place where they could no longer fight, neither physically nor mentally. The concepts of winning whilst appearing to lose, of interchanging truth and falsehood, and of becoming close to nature were all new to me. I certainly don't claim to have mastered these things, but this exposure, along with the distinct mindset that seems to go with the art, were to have a profound effect on me.

After an initial period of having to un-learn everything I had learnt in the Ju-Jitsu club (as it seemed at the time), my confidence quickly picked up. It was a different approach, with different ways of moving, and different goals. I liked it, and quickly started absorbing as much of the history and background as possible. I began to relax, mentally and physically, and move more naturally. I started to think less of 'having to win' when performing a technique, and began to flow. At least a little.

Around this time I was also absorbing a great deal of martial philosophy, both from senior figures within the Bujinkan (notably

Choose Life

Hatsumi Sensei and Stephen K. Hayes), and also from elsewhere, such as Sun Tzu, Musashi, Bruce Lee, Geoff Thompson and Peter Consterdine. Between the physical and mental aspects of the training itself, and the wide-ranging influences that I was studying outside the dojo, my own thinking began to change significantly.

Meanwhile, the training continued, and with it my techniques and grasp of the philosophical aspects grew. My confidence and self-belief were slower to develop, perhaps held back by the 'betrayal' of my previous experiences. I was always left doubting, although I may have been holding myself back with the constant questions of *what if, what if, what if?* Irrespective of the reasons, I didn't establish a convincing belief in my ability to cope with a real life violent encounter, which in time became part of my decision to leave the Bujinkan.

Others factors in this decision were on a psychological level. Although it had at first been a wonderful and free sensation to let go of the restricting discipline that was part and parcel of my previous art, I later felt that I was without discipline. I accepted that discipline had to be self-imposed, but this just wasn't working for me. Although I had gained much in terms of freedom, I had also lost something along the way. I stuck with it, blindly hoping that things would sort themselves out, but it wasn't to be. It became apparent that some of my needs would not be addressed within this art - a fact that wasn't going to go away, however much I wished it. My path was slowly but surely going in a different direction from the dojo and instructor that I had spent four great years with, and after some indecision on my side, we parted company. There were no bad feelings - in fact the instructor is still a good friend of mine - but it was time for me to change direction.

I had no plans, no alternatives, no other dojo lined up, but I knew this was still the right decision. Not rationally, but I just somehow knew. After trying very hard to think through my options and figure out where my future lay, I eventually realised this was not the right way to approach my situation. No good ever comes of trying to force the right decision, so instead I decided to surrender this to the flow of things, and accept that the next step would come to me when the time was right. And it did.

A few months on, and I came across a small Goshinkwai Combat club. First time on the mat and everything felt right, totally street orientated, and although it might be scruffy looking to the beginner, there was clearly a beautiful art just beneath the surface. Straight away I could see that I would be training with these guys for a long time to come. A few weeks later, and we started looking at the essence of the art - not the techniques themselves, but rather the spirit from within that actually makes the techniques work. Not just determination, but the inner strength, at times the anger that comes from the very core of your being. This is the thing that will make these techniques real, the thing that will actually bring you through a dangerous situation in one piece. The drills and exercises we did to focus this 'spirit' left me with a strange feeling in the pit of my stomach. Not just the blood-rush, not just the adrenalin - I was familiar enough with these to recognise that they were present, but so was something else. It was a very warm, very fluid feeling, and one that I found I could transmit outwardly with intention. I left that evening with a strange sensation in both my stomach and my heart, and knew with certainty that I had just turned a corner in my training. An exciting new chapter had begun, and things were never going to be quite the same again.

I am aware that this projection of spirit or intention will sound familiar to students of many different martial systems. The application taught within the Goshinkwai Combat system transmits the mental determination through the physical. This not only makes a physically powerful technique, but one that also shows (feels) your aura and determination on a psychological level. The feeling of overwhelming your opponent, of completely dominating him, is transmitted from (if not before) the first contact, and then continuously. This total and continuous domination then feeds through into the physical aspects of the technique.

So far, so good. But at the same time as giving out this continuous and overwhelming sense of domination, the physical body is able to relax. It can explode into action, relax and breathe, and then explode again, as required to complete the technique - this on/off switch helps to eliminate unnecessary tension in the body. And remember that whilst all of this is going on, we also continue to project the overwhelming mental domination. Easy to say, not too difficult to understand on the intellectual level, but actually this is not so easy to put into practice. For me it is particularly difficult to call-up this attitude from my hara (pit of the stomach) without becoming physically tense. Likewise I can remain relaxed, but then find it difficult to access and transmit this intensely powerful mental state. I have to say that there are certainly others who teach similar principles - no-one has copyright on this stuff after all - however, this was the first time I had trained with people who keep this high on the agenda. I have to say I was astounded by the impact of this, as it utterly changed every technique. Every single technique.

This experience had a huge impact on me, largely because of how it felt. Make no mistake about it, this is something that you have to feel in order to understand - feeling is believing, as someone once said. Once you have felt this, the truth becomes self-evident, and words of explanation are no longer necessary. Although I am only scratching the surface of this right now, I know that this has changed my entire world in terms of training.

What is more, is that this system has the potential to give the best of both my previous approaches, but without the drawbacks. The strength and discipline of old, but without the tension that came with it. The relaxation and movement of more recent times, but without the weakness of spirit. Finding once again the confidence of old, but now with the blinkers off, allowing the beginnings of some degree of honest knowledge and experience to flourish. It will undoubtedly take time for the doubts to go completely, as they can leave a very stubborn mark on the psyche. But they have already started to fade a little.

No longer is there an expectation that I will have to do battle with life. As well as having the confidence to expect not to fight (and therefore no longer creating unnecessary battles), I also have an increasing confidence to fight, should the need arise. These are different and complimentary sides of the same coin, which come together only from doing the right training, and putting the hours in. As I have said, the benefits of both previous approaches, without the negatives of either.

And most importantly of all - the self-belief is starting to come back. Only this time with a solid foundation.

14. Religion vs. Spirituality

My personal views on religion are fairly straightforward:

- **There is no such thing as a God.**
- **There is no afterlife.**
- **There is no heaven.**
- **There is no hell.**

This is not meant to offend anyone, these are just my honest beliefs.

If you take a look at the world's major religions, the main requirement is usually an unquestioning faith in a supreme being. Despite the common depiction of the benign shepherd and his flock, the relationship actually treats the believer as some sort of misguided child, and the deity as somewhere between an aloof parent and combined judge/jury/executioner. Gods are to be obeyed, sometimes feared or placated, but always in the name of love. Beliefs must be accepted and not challenged. Take man-made dogma and swallow it whole, even if you know if doesn't quite make sense. Most religion is heavily dependant on blind faith, and gives little in the way of personal responsibility. Hmmm, is it just me that smells a rat here?

I have no doubt that the majority of these religions have deeply significant spiritual teachings at their core, and the essence of those teaching will typically be love, peace and forgiveness. It's hard to argue with those as guiding principles, however they often get lost when these teachings are applied to our day to day lives.

Personally I care little whether someone believes in a God or not, much less which one. What is important to me is the person themselves, their nature, and their capacity to love and serve others. I also value an ability to see what is important in this world, and an intention to make a personal and positive contribution. Specific beliefs are hold little relevance to me - the real significance is in the way that people behave, the standards they hold in their hearts, and how the two match up. It also helps to understand whether this is a static position, or if they are continuing to grow and develop.

As this overlaps with many established religious beliefs, you might well ask what my problem is. Essentially I feel there is a huge gulf between religion and spirituality, and that religions generally don't do what it says on the tin. Leaving theological debate to one side for a moment, one of the main problems is that organised religion is just that - it is organised. The focus, despite what they might claim, is often different from the core spiritual teachings. The main drive might really be bums on seats, or knocking doors to spread the 'good word'. Once inside it might be more of a social club than anything, with more concern visible over who does what for the summer fete than about people's spiritual well-being. So many different churches, and although many in this country are offshoots from a single religion, even they can't quite agree on what is right, or how to best look after their 'flocks'.

What has been created - magnificent buildings, extensive written dogma, complex ceremonies and traditions - is all man made. Every religious or spiritual leader seems to consider themselves as being charged with spreading God's word, however they each use their own differing interpretations. I don't like to nitpick, but this is not God's word at all. Even if I accepted the existence of a God, this is Man's word. Not just the modern preacher's interpretation, but also the age-old passages that he is reading from - the 'holy text' is also the word of Man. All of it. Actually, the combined works of lots of Men. Usually at different times, often not quite agreeing with each other, and always putting their own slant on things, whether intentionally or otherwise. In itself, this will sometimes be harmless, and other times more purposeful. Let's stick with the harmless for the moment - for example, one branch of Christianity feels that a piece of bread is a symbol they do not need to use within their worship. Another denies that it is symbolic, and insists that it actually becomes Christ's flesh. Before you know it, we suddenly have irreconcilable differences between the two major versions of the Christian faith. Really? Given the state of the planet, in both physical and spiritual terms, I would have thought we might put our energies to more useful matters, if we were really concerned about saving Man's soul from the hot and fiery place. We'll be arguing about what colour hats to wear next...

And what of the not-so-harmless? How many wars have been fought in the name of a God? How many have died? How much suffering in this world has been caused in the name of religion? Sure, the people in your local church will say that this is an abhorrent misuse of God's name, but hey, that's not what the militants are saying, is it? What about *their* God, the one that's more *eye for an eye* than yours? What's wrong, has that one gone out of fashion? Next we might be saying that the 'fire and brimstone' God of the last century might not have been real. Wild accusations might follow about that version of God having been used to control the masses...

Despite my own beliefs, I don't wish like to sound as if I am just mocking. The plain fact is that the various religions have many hundreds of thousands of followers in the UK alone. Irrespective of what I might think, many people do want what is on offer. Or perhaps it is more accurate to say that they **need** what is on offer. Some people lack the strength and courage to stand up tall against the hardships of life, some need a spiritual or emotional crutch to lean on, and that's alright. Others need to feel that there is purpose in this cold universe, that everything happens for a reason, and is part of a master plan. Even if we can't understand that plan, it helps to know that the reasons are there somewhere, and that someone is looking after it all. This is understandably common among those who have suffered loss and tragedy. Others may just be weak by nature, and to be fair, it is better for them to be led by religious men who are (usually) positive influences, than by others who might lead them astray. Some have been brought up around a particular faith, grown up surrounded by these teachings, and will have accepted many so called 'fundamental truths' before being mature enough to question them. By the time you are old enough to know your own mind, the propaganda has done it's job, and you may never see past the brainwashing. This is no more than indoctrination under a different name.

To be honest, I don't really object to people's beliefs - if you need it, then you need it. And to be fair, there are worse things to become wrapped up in. Crazed militants aside, the world's major religions are generally both positive and harmless. I would never dream of telling anyone that they are wrong, because we are each leading our own lives, and after all, who am I to say? Come to think of it I wouldn't even tell them that there is a bigger picture to be seen. Not unless they asked.

There is also the fact that people will only see the plain truth of things when they are ready to. For example, it doesn't matter how many times I might tell you that the world is round, unless you are open to the fact that your previous beliefs might be flawed, that perhaps there might be another explanation - until you reach that point, your mind will be closed to my words. Rather than listening, you patiently wait for me to stop my misguided nonsense. Some might smile at my foolish beliefs, one or two might even mock my obvious stupidity - *ha ha, what an idiot. Everyone knows that we would all fall off...*

Although some of my views on religions are long-held, it is interesting to see that as I have become increasingly aware of the spiritual aspects of life, I have found myself moving even further away from organised religion. I come from a semi-religious background - my mum has been a regular church-goer throughout her life, something that continues to this day. When I have talked to her about some of my thoughts, especially around this separation of spiritual matters and church matters, I got a very different answer from that which I might have expected. She felt that if Christ were to return to earth today, he would be far from happy with much of what the churches have become. He would not like a deal of what is being practiced or preached, and would likely declare that many of the world's Christian/Catholic churches have lost their way from his teachings over two thousand years ago. With that, she smiled, as she pointed out that perhaps we are not quite so far apart in our thinking as we had always assumed. With that I smiled, also.

A friend of mine is a practising Muslim, and some years ago we talked about his faith, and how it provided a framework within which he could live - how it guided him, showed him how to behave, to become a better person and contribute positively to society. Throughout the conversation I found myself marvelling that the benefits of his faith were exactly those that I had found within the martial arts. Two unlikely sounding routes to the same thing perhaps, but we could both see the common ground. This is what I am looking for - the common factors at the core, the irrefutable truths. How we might reach them is all but irrelevant.

This was also picked up in *Heretic* - a novel by Bernard Cornwell. The main character in this excellent book was Thomas, the bastard son of a priest. The story was set in the fourteenth century, when the church virtually owned the souls of folk throughout the land, both high born and low. For a variety of reasons, unethical church leaders had decreed that Thomas was to be excommunicated - thrown out of the church, with his soul effectively cast asunder. Thomas was shocked beyond belief, and found it impossible to imagine life without God. For a man living in those dark ages, especially as the son of a priest, this was almost a sentence of death.

His companion had also been cast out as a heretic, however she felt no such despair. She explained that it doesn't matter if you are not allowed into the church, because that is not where God is - not the church as a building, nor as an establishment. Instead God is everywhere. Look for him in the fields, in the air and the trees - there is no need to prove his existence in these places, because we can all feel his presence.

On a spiritual level it is hard to disagree with the power of this presence, whatever name you might choose to give it. Try walking across the local park on a cold frosty morning as the bright sunlight is bringing everything to life. Try looking at the cycles of the changing seasons - so dulled by familiarity that we no longer see the detail, but look afresh and you will see undeniable magic, powerful forces at work. Look at the intricate complexities of food chains and eco-systems, there is a truly incredible life-force within each part, and also connecting it all together. There is something irresistible about this power, and when it touches us, we know the truth in our hearts - that we too are connected to this force.

For me, this incredible force goes by a simple name - Nature. And to be closer to Nature is something that we can all benefit from.

A couple of years ago I found myself taking a look at some Buddhist practices, in particular Mikkyo - The Japanese Diamond and Lotus Tradition. Prior to this I had always assumed (in my ignorance) that Buddhism was just another religion, however it turns out not to be the case at all. There is no god to be worshipped, in fact quite the opposite - in Buddhism we are asked to take responsibility for our own spirituality and growth, and encouraged to go out and look, question and examine everything, so that we can find the true path ourselves. As I have already mentioned, the characters such as Kongosatta and Fudo Myo-oh within this tradition are not there to be worshipped, rather they serve as positive representations of different aspects of the self, to be used as role models of a sort, to guide your thinking and behaviour, and help you to find the right qualities within yourself. Very different from 'religion', as this promotes a truth where everyone has all that they need to find spiritual enlightenment, already there within themselves. The journey then becomes a matter of peeling away layers, stripping bare, and polishing that which is inside.

A universal theme within Buddhism is the guidance known as the Four Noble Truths and the Noble Eightfold Path. Inevitably there are varying translations and interpretations, however I have reproduced the following from Stephen K. Hayes' thought provoking book 'Action Meditation', as I felt this truly captured the essence of these teachings.

The Four Noble Truths

i.   To the unenlightened mind, the experience of life is characterised by the anxiety of discontent.

ii.   Dissatisfaction with life comes from desiring to have what cannot be had, and desiring to avoid what cannot be avoided.

iii.   Since causes always generate results, and effects always follow causes, it is possible to overcome the discontented life orientation.

iv.   The way to overcome dissatisfaction is to let go of those mistaken views, habits and delusions that get in the way of clarity of spirit. The way to begin to cultivate clarity is to follow the Buddhist Noble Eightfold Path

Choose Life

I have found irrefutable truths within the words above, and am sure that you will be able to associate the essence of this with events/issues within your own lives. When I lose my way within the rush of daily life, I find it invaluable to come back to these words and use them to set myself back on to the right path.

Please read these points slowly and thoughtfully before moving on, as an understanding and acceptance of the Four Noble Truths is essential if you are to make good use of the Eightfold Path overleaf.

The Noble Buddhist Eightfold Path

1.   Proper View
Ultimate truth is ultimate truth - see life as it really is and stay tuned in!

2.   Proper Thought
Take charge of inner vision - set your mind on what you need to see!

3.   Proper Speech
Communicate truth - say what you need to hear!

4.   Proper Action
Work constructively - generate what you need to experience!

5.   Proper Livelihood
Take responsibility for what surrounds you in this world!

6.   Proper Effort
Keep your positive momentum going - make the right things happen!

7.   Proper Mindfulness
Use every moment as an opportunity to grow - everything matters!

8.   Proper Concentration
Consistent meditation - keep a centred spirit!

This is fantastic, and I would encourage you to give the above words some serious thought, as there is an incredible amount of power within them, just waiting to be discovered. This is not at odds with religious beliefs, and is a time proven way of focussing yourself on personal growth and development.

Personally I find the Buddhist mindset very refreshing and natural - it urges us to take responsibility for ourselves, and in doing so aims to set us free. However, as appealing as this may sound, it is also important to recognise that any systematic approach to meditation is essentially a teaching mechanism. It's fine in order to get seekers onto the path, point them in the right direction and gain some understanding, but ultimately all of this structure has to be left behind, otherwise it becomes just another self-limiting system. I don't doubt the universal truths within the teachings, but personally I need to take this away from the man-made structure, and apply it in a way that fits with my own approach to life. I need to be in a place where meditation is about my mindset when I'm walking the dog, rather than sitting in a silent room for two hours. I am much more of a pragmatist than a philosopher, and find a practical approach far more rewarding than investing huge amounts of time into sitting still, contemplating different aspects of life, or different faces of myself. I'm not knocking meditation - far from it, in fact this is something I intend to explore further for myself, as it seems an accepted fact that meditation has many, many positives from which we can benefit.

However, a word of caution...

Many years ago I trained with a guy called Ali, who in addition to our shared interest in the martial arts, was also getting hooked on meditation. To the extent of going on weekend meditation courses where (as far as I could see) you sat quietly in a room for two days. Hmm. To the extent that he was getting out of bed two hours early every day in order to have time to meditate. Hmm. Although it all seemed a bit strange to me, I was also deeply curious, as meditation is used by many on route to development and enlightenment. We had the same (superb) Ju-Jitsu Instructor at the time, a guy called John - one day the two of them were talking, and their conversation found it's way to the following question: *if you could be any person, from any part of history, who would you be?*

Ali began to talk about a group of monks that live and pray together in some desolate place or other. Very heavy on the meditation, as you might expect. However, within this group, there was one monk who made the others look like amateurs, in that he apparently spent all day, every day in a duck-shed within the monastery grounds, meditating. A short break or two for food and bodily functions, and then back into the duck-shed, back into his meditative state. Ali thought this was awesome, and felt that this was the person from history that he would most like to be.

John was smiling as he told this story, but it concerned me. It still does. Sure, I can understand the pull of such dedication, and I can certainly see why it might appeal to some, but at the end of the day, this guy spends his whole life in a duck-shed! I don't laugh out of ignorance - I can see that at an advanced level, the potential for sheer joyous rapture through meditation must be difficult to turn away from. Others who have been at such an advanced level have described this as having chains of gold - indescribable pleasures, but in the end, ones that must be given up if your growth is to continue.

This does rather sum up my dislike of the fragmented approach that we often have to personal growth. No matter how far this guy had come in his personal development, he became stuck along the way and was spending his days in a duck-shed. I'm sorry, but that isn't living - however wonderful your state of mind might become, it would be false. There are parallels here with using drugs to change your experiences in life - entirely possible, but if you go down this route then you are always in hiding from reality. In the story above, no matter what, you can never get away from the absolute truth that a man is living in a duck-shed. In my mind it is better to be a little less enlightened, but to put your knowledge to good use in this world. As powerful as meditation might be, it is ultimately a technique to be used, rather than an end in itself. Theory and exercises are but a starting point. Real life application is everything.

For years I have tried all sorts of different things, including breathing exercises, Junan Taisho stretching, and Tai Chi style exercises. The trouble, however, is that I am always left knowing that it isn't quite right for me. This is often accompanied by a vague but uncomfortable feeling that perhaps I just lack the required discipline. Although this was undoubtedly true on occasion, I can now see the main reason for this problem - all of the methods I had tried were focussing on specifics, when what I really needed was the whole picture, the whole of the elephant, if you like. I don't want to spend forty years in deep study of all the requisite parts, before hopefully being able to put them together. The real point is to learn now, and develop the strength of character to apply these lessons to my life as I go along. See the effect, assess the results, and continue to learn and adjust things as I carry on along my path. This has an immediate impact, starts improving my quality of life from day one, and continues to do so with each step taken. Much better than waiting until I have the perfect theoretical mindset, and then realising I'm eighty-five years old and need help getting to the toilet.

I will undoubtedly keep on learning throughout the course of my life - who knows, I might even end up a wise old man! But let's forget about the future, after all we build it through our actions in the present. Instead let us concentrate on making life better now, for all of us, and then we really can enjoy the journey. It is our spirit, and therefore our spirituality that is central to our continued growth - this is what enables us to overcome barriers and become more balanced people, and helps us to make an increasingly positive contribution to this world. Although this spirituality is to be found within most religions, there is usually a distinct lack of practical advice on how we might successfully apply it to our real lives.

And as for the rest of it? Who cares about the guy in the big hat with all of the ornate trappings - is that really necessary to transmit spiritual teachings? I think not. The important thing is that we all keep learning, and keep applying what we have learnt, for then we will be making this world a continually better place for those around us. And as a result, for ourselves. I may not be a religious man, but I do believe that we are all spiritual people - so let us strive for a fulfilling life **before** death.

15. Goal Setting

So what's the next step? It's a good question, and one that is not always so easy to answer. If you can see value in the issues discussed so far, if you have been bold enough to take a look at your own life and give some thought as to what is good, and what could do with some work - then what exactly are you are going to do next?

Perhaps you weren't thinking of doing anything, perhaps this has been interesting, but *hey, I'm not sure I'm ready to take any big steps just yet.* Fine, if this is what you want - sit tight and carry on exactly as you are. And try not to do too much harm to those around you in the meantime. This of course would be the same cop-out as my friend Ian made a few chapters ago, and to turn your back at this stage would be worse than ignorance, it would be a wilful choice. A decision to pretend that you aren't aware of the responsibility you hold for your own life, that you aren't aware of the sheer scale of your potential. And all because it feels a bit uncomfortable. If you are perfectly happy, getting enough of those moments of clarity and finding more contentment than aggravation in your day to day life, then fine. If not, I guess you always reserve the right to stick your head back in the sand, and that might even seem like the easier option. But things have changed. Last time, maybe you didn't know what else to do, maybe you couldn't see anything of the proverbial bigger picture, or didn't even know that there was one. Maybe you didn't know that you can take some degree of control, that starting to steer yourself in the right direction can actually be quite easy. Perhaps you stuck your head in the sand without knowing any of these things. However, it is more likely that you knew things weren't right, that carrying on regardless wasn't an answer, and that there must be more to life. It can be difficult to break out from this, and you may not have felt sure that you were supposed to. Or even allowed to.

But now you know. Now you can see that not only is this within your power, but it is also as straightforward as you decide to make it. And now that you **do** know a little better, now that you **are** aware of there being other ways, sticking your head back in the sand is no longer an easy option. And if you did, then all of this would be going around and around inside your head, reminding you of the truth.

A small but vitally important point about reading this book, or perhaps attending a seminar, watching a film or anything else that motivates or inspires you, is that you must take action. You must do something as a result, and do it quickly, whilst the enthusiasm is still with you. It's all too easy to put off until next week, next month, or next year, but by then this is all a distant memory, and the energy that came with the initial rush of enthusiasm has long since left. It is vital that you act now, before it becomes impossible once more. And if you don't? Then this whole thing is reduced to having been merely an 'interesting' experience. Nothing less, but certainly nothing more.

So how do we move on from here? What is it that you are going to do? One of the most positive steps forward is to set goals for yourself. This works on a number of levels - in the first place, if you don't know what it is you are setting out to achieve, how can you ever achieve it? And how would you know if you did succeed? Stating the obvious perhaps, but without a goal your well intentioned efforts are likely to be misdirected. When you set yourself well balanced goals, you can see for yourself that you are already starting to take positive steps, just by clarifying your intentions. As a result this gives you a feeling of purpose and progress, and a sense of excitement at moving forwards. The drive and energy that comes with this can be put back into yet more action, then suddenly you're away, and building some real positive momentum!

There can also be one or two problems associated with goals, specifically with the details. For example - setting too many goals, setting goals that are too easy or too difficult, or failing to put timescales on your aims. Any of these can be enough to stop even the most determined person in their tracks within a week or two.

The biggest trap I fell into was that of creating over-elaborate plans. After all, when you realise how slack you've been, and have identified all of the areas that you need to improve, then it becomes easy to feel you must incorporate each and every one of these into your new plan, in order to become the 'new you'. I did this about a year ago, with the poorly defined aims of becoming more relaxed, less stressed, and to have a generally healthier lifestyle. I picked a few things I should be doing less of, a few that I should be doing more of, and figured that if I got about six or seven of these right each day, then I would be on the right track. To firm my resolve I then drew up a plan for the first month that looked like this, with the thought of putting ticks against everything that I was successful with each day:

Day	No Coffee	No Fried Food	No Sugar	No Alcohol	Drink Lots Water	Eat Fruit	Stretch-ing	Strength Exercises	Martial Arts Training	Total
1	√	√	-	√	√	√	√	√	-	7
2	√	√	-	√	√	-	√	-	√	6
3	-	-	√	-	-	-	√	√	-	3
4	√	-	-	-	√	-	-	-	-	2
5	-	-	-	√	√	√	-	-	-	3
6	-	√	-	-	-	-	-	-	-	1
7	-	-	√	-	-	-	-	-	√	2
8	√	-	√	√	-	-	√	√	-	5
9	-	√	-	-	-	-	-	√	-	2
10	-	√	-	-	-	-	-	-	-	1
etc										

In the first couple of days my 'performance' was artificial simply because I knew that I was monitoring it. This was positive at first, as it prompted me to do more of the good things, but then I started to slip back into my old ways. Not only was there too much for me to concentrate on, I also had a chart to fill in. One that would give me two or three out of nine for the day, and make me feel lousy. Bad enough that in my heart I already knew I was failing my new regime, without having it proved to me statistically. This didn't give me the drive I needed to make my new programme work, instead it made me feel guilty, and then quite low about the abject failure that I could now *prove* myself to be.

Of course this fell apart long before the end of the first month. It was overcomplicated, and saw me spreading myself so thin that I couldn't focus successfully on any one part, let alone the plan as a whole. It all came crashing down, although at the time I didn't realise that I'd actually set myself up to fail.

During one of my sessions with the Counsellor, she pointed out that the first step in any plan of action does not have to be the perfect starting point, or even necessarily address all of the issues. I must confess, I looked at her as if she was barking mad. She went on to explain her thoughts - because I was so determined that I must take the right steps, I had become incapable of taking any actions at all, as I was so uncertain whether they were the 'right' ones. Rather than being concerned over exactly what to do, or precisely how to do it, the Counsellor suggested that I should just start, make myself take even one or two small actions and then review my progress. It might even turn out to be the wrong action, but it wouldn't matter, the point is that you start the ball rolling, getting off your arse and actually doing something. This gives some movement, some positive action, and a feeling of putting yourself back in the driving seat. Whether the first step is a great one or not, you will have broken out of the resigned apathy, and given yourself some momentum that you can build upon.

Going back to the ridiculous programme I had set for myself, a better approach would have been to look at which of these many goals were the most important. Had I done this, I would probably have decided that it would have been the drinking. At the time I would have been happy if I could have abstained from alcohol for a month, and this would have been a much simpler and more achievable goal. As for the others, well, general issues around health are easier to pick up when you are not drinking, so some of the other points would have followed naturally, but without the need for an over-the-top programme.

A goal of giving up alcohol for a month is straightforward enough to define, however some goals can be more difficult to pin down. There are different ways of setting goals, but the most common method by far is that of 'SMART' objectives. This is usually mentioned in conversation by people trying to prove they know a thing or two, who will then laugh as if to say *what clap-trap, what nonsense, what management bullshit*. This type of attitude however, is no more than a display of ignorance. In fact, the SMART approach to setting goals and objectives is as effective as it is simple. Basically the letters stand for the following:

Specific
Measurable
Achievable
Realistic
Timescales

S-M-A-R-T. Geddit?

For a goal to be properly set, then you need to be specific about what it is you want to achieve. There needs to be a way of measuring progress/achievement, or else you won't know when you have achieved your goal. Worse, you might not be able to tell how you are progressing on route - a sure-fire motivation killer. Your goal must also be achievable, and realistic. Yes, it is good that a goal stretches you, but if you set your sights too high too soon, then you are setting yourself up to fail - something to be avoided at all costs. Finally, it must include definite timescales, otherwise you will have a never ending target, making it too easy to delay starting, or to put your goal to one side as soon as the going gets tough.

For example, suppose I was a recreational runner (now we are stretching the imagination to breaking point). Perhaps I regularly go for a jog in the morning before work, around a mile, mile and a half. If it was a real desire of mine to improve my fitness, build my stamina and self-discipline, then I might decide to set myself a goal. It could look like one of these:

I will do more running in the New Year
or
I will run further than before
or
I will run faster than before, and further when I can

This is exactly the sort of goal that will do nothing for you. This won't help in any way, as there is nothing specific about it. More running? Well, how much more? More times a week, or a greater distance? What about running further? Well, how much further? A mile? A yard? The question you need to ask yourself is this - **exactly** what is it that you want to do? As I've already said, if you don't know, then you can be certain that you won't achieve it. So perhaps I would like to run quite a long way - let's say ten miles. Tall order...? Well, maybe, but lets apply the SMART theory to this.

We're already fairly specific, although we haven't thought about how quickly I might cover the ten miles. After all, I'm sure I can do it in about four or five days... Perhaps I might be happy if I could cover this in a couple of hours. So that's to run ten miles within two hours - specific enough for me. By nature this particular target is easily measurable, both in terms of distance and time, so that's the 'S' and the 'M' covered. But what about the rest of it?

Achievable, Realistic, Timescales....
It seems to me that in this example, these three are tied together - that is to say that how achievable this is, and how realistic it might be, is largely down to the timescales that I choose for myself. If I were to attempt to run this distance by the end of the week, then clearly I would fail, as it will take much more of a build up than this. So perhaps this is a six month goal. I could do this in less time, or extend it, and this is where I need to balance how much I want to achieve my goal, against the time and effort I can put in. A common mistake at this point is to over-extend yourself - not always a bad thing, but when the initial rush of enthusiasm passes, we can often feel that we've bitten off more than we can chew. In turn this gives us an 'acceptable' excuse to pack it all in when the motivation starts to drop. So, common sense and moderation weighed against commitment - lets go with the six months. What does my goal look like now?

> *I will complete a ten mile run within two hours, by the end of a six month period (insert date)*

This is a well defined goal. I would know if I achieved this, and would easily be able to match progress in training against both the distance and the timescales set out. You can create your own goals, and apply the SMART theory in a similar manner.

To take another angle on this, a phrase I came across recently is 'Fulfilling our Potential'. This is a fairly modern phrase, often used in connection with education i.e. *I would like my children to be able to fulfil their potential.* A noble thought, and one that contains an essential understanding - recognising that potential is individual for each of us. No doubt understood by generations of educators, however not necessarily as obvious to the rest of us. In fact it often seems that others achieve more because they are able to, because they get the life chances, the lucky breaks and so on. And where others seem to have been blessed with a better starting position than our own, it's easy to decide that there is no point in trying. But this couldn't be more wrong - we all have a great deal of potential irrespective of our background, or how far we have already come. With this in mind, don't be daunted if you are taking the first tentative steps of your journey, this should be exciting and exhilarating - after all, you have the most to gain!

When we talk of potential in terms of children, although it is often about academic achievement, it is generally slanted in terms of *enabling* children to meet their full potential – i.e. it is usually aimed at the parents, teachers etc. who are in a position to influence this, rather than directly at the child themselves. Of course this can often work extremely well to support our children, but what about us 'grown-ups'? How many of us have fulfilled our potential, even in just one or two aspects of our lives? Do you know any that have? If you do, then I would guess that you can count them on the fingers of one hand. Probably the fingers of one finger. Doesn't seem right, does it...?

When you step into your role as a man or woman of this world, then you take responsibility for your whole life - your safety, your health, wealth, employment, living arrangements, personal relationships, eating and drinking habits, paying the bills, doing the shopping... the list is an endless one. More than you ever realised as a kid, but hey, this is the price of freedom. Somewhere amongst all this, lost without reference, is the fact that you also became responsible for your own development, the journey towards meeting your own individual potential. By now, there is no-one else looking out for you on this score (unless you are really lucky), so the first thing is for you to recognise this loss. In truth, most of us are so wrapped up in the whirlwind of work, home, family and the sort of chores listed above, that we don't ever stop to draw breath, let alone take time to reflect. We charge on, always at full speed, hoping to hang on until we can crash out at home with a take-away and a DVD, or go drown ourselves in beer at the pub. But when do we actually stop, when do we take a step outside of our lives and think?

I stopped, just recently, and found myself wondering about the practicalities of this. Fulfil our potential...? It's quite easy to say, but actually isn't this just too big and formless to take on? How the hell do you get a grip on something as monstrously huge as this, not to mention vague...? It's no good preaching about these things if I can't work it out for myself. So let's give it a try.

My own potential? Hmm, well I'm not doing too badly, but I do seem to be at a bit of a standstill. There is just never enough time, and that seems to be a common theme for us all. Not enough hours in the day, not enough days in the week - as problems go, I guess it's straightforward enough. But then again, perhaps it's not. After all I've got the same amount of time as anyone else - twenty four hours a day, seven days a week, fifty two weeks a year... so maybe it's how I choose to use it. Remember though, that much of it is filled with work, family commitments or unavoidable chores... hmmm, not making headway here. Hang on, what about the evenings - there's often a bit of time there... oh yeah, but I'm always too knackered to be bothered. Can't expect me to do anything creative when I'm exhausted every night.

Ahh, so it's not just about time, it's also that I'm usually exhausted. A lack of energy translates quickly into a lack of enthusiasm, the self-discipline fails, confidence vanishes, and apathy sets in. So this really is about having the energy. Interesting...

The next question is more obvious - what impacts on my energy? Obviously alcohol - much as it seems to be a treat at the time, it does leave you listless the next day (at least). What else? The greasy food, the caffeine, the sugar intake - thought I'd sorted the last two, but they've crept back in with a vengeance when I wasn't looking. Then there's the negative attitude, failing morale and self-belief. Not to mention self-esteem. I'm not doing any exercise either, not even walking the dog regularly - I seem to have almost stopped doing this too.

I spoke in an earlier chapter about the role of alcohol, but here a different relationship starts to appear - I'm looking at the same picture, but starting to see different patterns. So, take an evening when I have a few beers or a bottle or wine - do I use that time to do anything positive or productive? No, because I am settling down to 'enjoy' a drink. Exercise obviously doesn't go hand in hand with this... What about decent food? Lettuce or carrots are hardly going to the most likely option for snack time after a few cans of Stella or a bottle of red, so it's always going to be something unhealthy. I'll probably become dehydrated during the evening, and then there's the next day - even more dehydrated. Likely to be running late in the morning, so I would pick up a bacon and egg on route to work. Coffee to get me going, more coffee to keep me going - don't bother with water because I need a stronger fix. Even more coffee. And sugar. Negativity - partly because it seems to come along with the poor diet, but also because I'm aware that the crap that I'm taking into my body is a short term fix, but a long term problem. I feel stuck in a cycle of increasingly unhealthy living. This is worse because I know that I should know better, in fact I know that I **do** know better, so I feel pretty low about the whole thing. Not good.

So what to do? The common thread here is the alcohol. Not just for the obvious reasons, but take this out, and see what happens. I feel brighter in the morning, and don't need the coffee. Drink some water, have time to take the dog for a quick walk and I can hear the birds, see the trees and feel the air. Then it's off to work, but I've already had a bit of toast and don't fancy the greasy butty. Drinking mainly water, perhaps with the odd cup of tea, but no coffee fixes, and no sugar snacks. Energy, energy, energy. Until the next evening comes around with the next few beers...

The Homer Simpson part of me wants to object at this point, but you can easily see a clear path from here, one that deals with the excessive alcohol intake and genuinely seems to hit all of the other issues along the way. Get this one under control and we might see me being more relaxed, less stressed, with a reasonable diet, and feeling better in body and mind. As a result I would then be well placed to really start moving towards my potential.

So, time to set a goal for myself? Yes, and of course it comes back to the double act of stress and alcohol. Neither of which are good for me, both of which have an adverse effect on my life in general, and my loved ones in particular. No point in coming this far without dealing with this, is there? I've ducked this one for long enough - now that I can see it for what it is, it's time to take some real action. Not only real, but sustainable. Absolutes don't seem healthy - to never drink again is unrealistic, and also likely to fail when the enforced self discipline cracks. Anyhow, isn't strict abstinence just another form of excess? Haven't we already said that such strict self-control is unnecessary? This is not the way to live, at least not for me. Enforced abstinence can be a holding point, but to move on we need to bring this back to the context of my whole life. My own personal bigger picture.

So the answer becomes self-evident, and can be written as a goal. One which is not only specific, but measurable. And one that can be made realistic and achievable by being sensible about the timescales. Let's have a go, shall we:

> *I will not drink any alcohol for the purpose of reducing my stress levels, until the end of the month.*

It is only the second day of the month today, so this gives me a good four weeks. I can drink for social reasons (no more than a couple of times a week), but **not** because of stress. The implication here is that I will have to find alternative ways of dealing with the stress. Although I have a good idea what many of these will turn out to be, I don't need to define them, let alone set them as goals. In general I might drink more water or do more exercise, and when I feel stressed I might hit the punch bag, walk the dog, or do whatever. What works for me on one day might not on another, so I will need to be flexible in my use of coping strategies. By setting myself one simple goal I can keep this in mind, but still be able to allow myself a can of beer or glass of wine with my wife or friends. And it's good to be able to enjoy a couple of beers for the right reasons, instead of drinking like it's some sort of race. Of course there is the risk here that I might slip-up, and start guzzling again whilst pretending it's just social drinking. But there is always one person that will know the truth. Me. And I can never really hide from that.

So that's my goal, to be reviewed at the end of the month, or earlier if need be. What about yours? What is your starting point?

In the past I always felt that having personal goals was somewhat selfish. After all, my real goal is to be the best I can be for my family. The best father I can be. The best husband I can be (granted I may still have some work to do here!). Because of this, it seemed that having other 'lower' goals of my own would be difficult. For example, I used to feel that if I wanted to become a writer, then this would involve many hours of isolated work, which would take me further away from my family, and therefore would not contribute towards making me a better father/husband. As much as I might have liked to work towards this goal for myself, I felt it would be selfish and counter productive when set against my 'higher' aims and ideals. It is only recently that I have been able to see past this - in fact becoming a writer has been a fantastic journey for me. My own personal growth has accelerated tremendously since I started to write, and the impact on my family has been positive. Although it is true that I have taken hours to write, I have organised this around my family as best I can, to minimise the impact. In any event, I know that I am a better person for developing in this way, and as a result I am better placed to be a good father and husband.

There is a balance to be found, because as noble as it might feel to be completely dedicated to others and take nothing for yourself, in the end it does you no good. And what is no good for you will invariably have a negative impact on those around you. Besides, if you don't value yourself at all, then why should anybody else?

So think of something that you want to do, and write it down. Then go get started. Come back to it in a few weeks and see what progress you've made. If it's nothing, then you will know why - you might procrastinate to others, but you know the truth yourself. And if you have done nothing towards achieving your goal, then try writing a smaller goal as a first step, and make the timescales shorter, so that you need to act straight away.

There is nothing you can't do, but in order to get this thing moving, you **must** do something positive for yourself. And start now

16. Higher Or Lower?

It sounded like I'd got the drinking thing sorted, didn't it? Except that it didn't work. It never does. Going from being on my knees again, to finding a 'magic fix' in the shape of setting a simple goal, just seemed too good to be true. And it was...

The problem here wasn't the goal I had set - the SMART process actually works very well. It's just that in this particular case I wanted so badly to find a solution which would allow me to continue drinking in some way, that my motives became skewed. When you want something so much, it's easy to pull the wool over your own eyes, to kid yourself that you're in control. That's exactly what I did with this goal of 'not drinking to relieve stress' - it might sound plausible enough, but unfortunately didn't address the underlying issue, the fact that I never did have control over my drinking habits. Whether the twenty-something weekend binge-artist, or the thirty-something home-drinker, I have never had control, and what's more, I don't know that it's possible, don't know that I can ever enjoy social drinking without going overboard.

It dawned on me recently that heavy drinkers often die in their early fifties - I can think of a number of well known examples of this. If I carry on drinking like this, then I've only got another dozen years or so left in me. Twelve years - my youngest would have just turned twenty, watching her old man going into the ground, way ahead of his time. Shit, with that perspective, I definitely have to stop. I don't want my wife and kids to be without me prematurely just because I'm an arse that can't stop pouring gallons of beer down my neck.

The trouble is that I really can't stop. Despite all of this I just carry on, racing towards disaster, and I can't cut down or stop. What the hell should I do? I was right earlier, I really am fucked. Despite all the growth and development, despite the incredible journey that I have found myself on, if I can't find a way through this, then it will all have amounted to nothing more than a slow suicide. In my frustration I continue to drink, heavier than ever now that I have admitted to myself that I have a problem. *Hey, if I've got a real problem then I must **have** to drink loads, right?* So I do.

The warning bells in my head are getting louder with each day that passes, I can see the big, sand-filled timer of my life draining away at twice the normal speed. Very unsettling. So I ignore it and start to think, to search in the hope that I can find a solution before this finally screws everything up for good. Sooner or later something will give - the odds are that it will either be my family or my sanity. Talk about a rock and a hard place...

I have no ace up my sleeve, no new ideas to save the day, so instead I go back to the stretching and the walking. Trying to relax enough to find the flow. I look once again at the hundreds of books on the shelf labelled *Mind/Body/Spirit*, desperately looking for the golden ticket, the magic formula that will wipe all of this from the record and let me get on with my new life. After a few days the initial panic subsides, and my vision starts to clear. I stop trying so hard, and then I remember - all of these different practices and techniques that are deemed to be answers, sold to us as solutions - aren't these just different starting points on the same journey, different parts of the same elephant?

Realising that I'm too close to the problem, and that once again I am trying too hard, I take several steps back until I can see the bigger picture once more. There has to be another way, one that is holistic rather than just breaking it all down into parts. Sure, all of the separate components have some validity, but if the quest is for a whole and fulfilling life, then breaking it down is only of use to find a starting point. Once we have this, and gain a degree of momentum, then we need to leave all of the component parts behind, if we are to find a way forward. A way that bring together that which is positive, but without the man-made rules, divisions and fixed methodologies.

A good example of this is the concept of karma - it has been said that this can be seen as a bank balance or credit card statement. Your actions, good or bad, are ultimately totted up, and you are either found to be in credit, or have to pay the price for being in debt. In this way, your actions in this life, positive or negative, come back to you. Personally I like the idea - in fact I think there are undoubtedly some truths in this. However it does not explain why someone is struck down by serious illness, or why a child dies so young - these dreadful things are without reason. Don't mistake the Universe as something that is either caring or malicious, it is simply cold. The world just keeps on turning, even if yours seems to be over. That may seem harsh, but it is also true. Terrible things do happen in this life, and many of us have reason to grieve, and ask *why, why, why?* Unfortunately there are easy no answers to this. As a close friend once said to me, *'If you accept what is, it is. If you don't accept what is, it is.'*

If you have been faced with tragedy in your life, then the plain truth is that there are no reasons or answers to ease your pain, unless you find yours within the blind faith of religion.

The principle of karma does however seem work on a personal level, in terms of our relationships with other people, and our emotional well-being. In this respect, we do all ultimately get what we deserve. Whether we can see this for ourselves is another matter, but the principles are sound - you do indeed reap exactly what you sow. What you give out to others is undoubtedly what you receive in return, what will shape your life and also those touched by your life. Positive leads to positive, negative leads to negative, no question.

Having said that, there is also something not quite right here. The notion that some sort of cosmic being is checking out your balance sheet, weighing up and deciding whether you deserve a good future or otherwise? Perhaps there is a demi-god up there in the clouds someplace, checking out little Johnny's record? *Oohh look, he's been mean to those two kids in his class – let's send some bad karma his way, that'll teach him...* This doesn't ring quite true, does it..?

My view is that the above notion of karma is essentially a teaching tool - the principles behind it are sound, and if it helps people to get on the right path, then there is no harm in it. But the truth is more simple. You do influence the way that people act towards you by the way that you interact with them - fairly obvious, we all want to be treated reasonably don't we? Taking this further, the way that you treat others and behave in general has a huge influence on yourself. Although this happens in the subconscious for most people, you are continually influencing yourself with good deeds and bad. Perhaps it is more accurate to describe this as being that which is positive and genuinely life enhancing, both for yourself and others; and then those actions and thoughts that are negative and go against life, health and well-being. You are the centre of your universe in this respect, and have a bigger influence on yourself than anyone or anything else.

For example, if I continue to behave in negative ways, even small ways, then this has a profound effect on me. Perhaps I continue to drink excessively in order to provide a release from life's pressures. Perhaps I eat junk food every day, or comfort-eat whilst watching TV in the evenings. Perhaps I cheat or lie to make my life easier - I might add a couple of extra items onto an otherwise genuine insurance claim, I could add a few extra miles on my mileage claim at work - I mean, where's the harm? Who's to know? Well, actually I'm to know. Irrespective of what I say, how I feel, or whether I claim to care or not, there is a simple bottom line. I know what is right and wrong, I know what is positive and what is negative. This is not about traditional moral values, but the real-life effect of your actions. In fact, the impact comes not from the actions themselves, but the motives and intentions behind them. It isn't always wrong to lie, perhaps you might be preventing someone's feelings from being hurt. It isn't always wrong to fight, perhaps you are protecting your family from harm. It all depends on your motivation - if the reasons why you act are genuine, positive, and not self-serving, then your actions, and therefore the consequences of those actions will also be positive. It is important to understand that this doesn't just mean the consequences for others, for the world around you - this also means the consequences for yourself.

There is a very real impact on your personal growth here, on your spiritual development. If you are looking to grow and improve your quality of life, then this has a massive impact, far beyond just 'holding you back'.

It is possible for you to continue growing and developing, irrespective of this. You can read books, talk to people, watch TV programmes or DVDs that motivate and inspire you, and I would of course recommend this to anyone. You can take some of the ideas and apply them to your life, make them work for you, improve your relationships, be a better mum or dad, a better partner or whatever. You can do all of this, and again I would recommend that you do so. But…

If you don't stop the negatives, then what follows is a mass of frustration and confusion. One so overwhelming that it can lead you to question all of your progress so far, all of the ideals you have adopted. It can even make you feel like turning your back on the whole thing, as what was once a positive and inspiring drive to improve yourself, now seems to have become a nonsense. What was once your salvation, the thing that kept you going through the difficult times, now seems to have become part of the problem, and is actually creating stress and anxiety. You know it doesn't make sense, especially when you thought that you'd come so far, but what was once a solution is now definitely looking like a problem.

So we go back to the drinking, and I'm still low. Not sure how I can get up off my knees, let alone get through this one. My common sense hasn't completely abandoned me yet, I still understand the rationale, and I know that if it was someone else, then I would want to shake them and shout *HEY, you know what the score is here, you have so much to gain here, but you will lose everything if you don't get up and take some bold action.* I am painfully aware of this, but I still can't get up. Maybe we crossed the line between stress and depression someplace back, and I never noticed. That doesn't help though, it's a bit like the self-fulfilling prophesy that came from admitting a drink problem - if I'm depressed as well, then I must **really** be struggling…

A day or two pass in limbo. In sheer frustration, I pose the question on an internet message board. I briefly explain that although I can stop drinking, it always creeps back, always builds back up, and I seem powerless to stop this dreadful cycle. I ask if anyone out there has been in the same position. I wasn't sure if anyone would answer, but I desperately hoped so. I needed help or advice from someone who really understood where I was, a voice of experience to point me in the right direction. Otherwise I would have to accept that all of my work, effort and progress had been for nothing, and this seemingly impassable wall really was the end of my journey. A few hours later and I have a couple of replies. The first talks about daily exercise being the key to well-being and self-discipline. No argument from me, the guy was right, but unfortunately I had slipped further down the slope than he could relate to, and this wasn't going to help me. A year ago this would have been good, sound advice. But not now.

The second reply suggests a book. I probably wouldn't have bothered, but he has included a link to the relevant page on Amazon. Even I can click on a link, and there it is... Easy Way to Control Alcohol by a guy called Allen Carr. I read the online reviews, hmm - some controversy? It looks interesting though - the author claims that you can stop drinking without any difficulty, without any withdrawal, and without any desire to drink again! That might sound unlikely, but it's only a few quid, got to be worth a look, hasn't it?

Two days later and it drops through the letter box. Reading the opening pages, I feel some disbelief. As I read further, the disbelief changes to a feeling that I am about to experience something life changing. The author explains that we are not in possession of the full facts, and that alcohol is dangerously misrepresented throughout Western society. In the first instance, the nature of alcohol as a poison is explored, comparing it first with nicotine, and then with heroin. Seems a bit harsh, but then again we all know that the stuff isn't exactly a health tonic, and overindulgence is obviously bad for us. But then you have to weigh this against the positives, as it often helps us to relax, to relieve stress, sometimes helps us to feel more confidant - Dutch courage and all of that. And let's not forget that I actually enjoy the taste. Ok, I've occasionally had some of the strong stuff that might have been a bit rough, but I definitely love a nice cold Stella or two. Or six. When the book starts to explore the 'brainwashing' aspect of how alcohol is portrayed, it even challenges the issue of taste. Ha! I know beyond any possible doubt that despite any misunderstanding or 'brainwashing', I definitely enjoy a nice cold beer - especially a Stella. With this in mind, I continue to read.

The book asks if you remember your first drink. Chances are it was something sweet - a bottle of cider, a glass of Perry or something similar. Despite the true taste being masked by a high sugar content, did it actually taste nice? Come to think of it - no. Actually it was awful, but like most of us I pretended to enjoy it, or at least not to mind, as this was adult stuff. None of us would have admitted to preferring a milkshake or a coke, those things were strictly for kids. So in the interests of behaving like adults, we kept on drinking the stuff and pretending to like it. After a while you get to the point where you believe that to be true, and then you're away...

So far there are many things in this book that are a revelation, that make perfect sense and have already started to change how I see alcohol. Strange then to have got this point about taste so very, very wrong. So I decide to try it out - eight cans of ice-cold Stella, more than enough for a taste test. Kid are safely tucked up in bed, and we're ready to go. It's like my usual evening drink, but with a difference - as I already know that it tastes damn good, when I let my taste buds **really** savour it then I will know for certain that the theory in this guy's book is flawed.

First can opened, nice big swig, but then instead of swallowing it straight down the hatch, I roll it around my mouth. All around, over my tongue a couple of times. Yuucch - what was that? My beloved Stella has the foulest taste - uurrgghh, there must be something wrong with it. Try another mouthful, just the same. I start to think there really must be something wrong with it, and take a normal swig, just to check. Straight down the throat, ahh, that's more like it, even if the first two have left a nasty taste in there. Hang on a minute, if there's nothing wrong with the beer, and I have just made sure to really taste it, swill around my mouth for a few seconds before swallowing, then what does that mean... *(dawning realisation)* ... shit, the book was right! I have conditioned myself, and also been conditioned by the adverts, by the idea of what drinking is supposed to be, and by everyone else acting along to the same script. Doesn't anyone think to question this? Arrgghh - this is my favourite drink, has been for about 15 years, and the first time I slow down enough to taste it properly, I find it is absolutely foul. Suddenly I can relate to the description of alcohol as poison. Suddenly my mind has been blown wide open...

Exactly how can I continue to drink after this? The book went on to expose various other myths around drinking, all the so-called 'benefits'. Even the overwhelming urge to keep on drinking that I have always described as 'having my drinking head on'. All of it untrue. This was absolutely mind blowing - one of those moments in your life that you never forget, the layers of reality folding back in on themselves. The next day I finish the book, follow their recommended ritual for a 'last ever drink' and am finished with it. For good.

You might expect immediate problems or strains - perhaps the shakes, or at least some mood swings. Definitely the craving, definitely that overwhelming, all-consuming urge to get absolutely bladdered. Or if not, then surely the quiet insistence that *one or two drinks will be ok, can't do you any harm…*?

Surprisingly not the case. Far from having the urge to drink, I am utterly relieved that I *don't have to drink.* Rather than feeling like a drinker who is going through a period of enforced abstinence, I actually feel glad to have put this behind me. Pleased, relieved, excited even to be approaching life afresh for the first time. I don't feel any need for alcohol in my life - this is rather strange for me as I have always been a drinker, and always known that I would remain this way for the duration. I am possibly the least likely person of all to go tee-total - friends and family are going to have a hard time believing this. It feels like I have stepped outside the boundaries of my life, and where I expected to find a desolate wasteland, I've actually found another version of my life, and it's somehow brighter and more colourful. If I can stop drinking and be happy with it, not just happy but **happier**, then anything is possible. Suddenly I'm living in a brave new world full of potential, full of exciting possibilities. Ironically it's the same world I always lived in, but it looks so incredibly different when the blinkers come off.

However evangelical I might be starting to sound, there really is a freedom that comes with this. Now that I have been given a realistic perspective, I am staggered to think how blind I was for so many years, how blinded most of the population are by the cultural myths and corporately funded brainwashing that is presented as 'normal'. Unbelievable. You may not want to give up drinking, as we tend to see this as one of the few pleasures we have, but then again I'm not telling you to give up. For me, it's enough that I don't drink. However, if you have ever wondered about the degree of control you actually have over your drinking, then I would say this book is essential reading. Worst case is that it doesn't ring true for you, but it's not like you have anything to lose. On the other hand there is much to be gained - few books are genuinely life changing, but this one certainly is.

Mind blowing as it was for me, this was again little more than taking another perspective, another view of the same mountain - although without the guidance of Allen Carr's amazing book I could never have seen it for myself. But the reality was that not only had I stopped drinking, I didn't want to drink either. I remained relieved for several weeks that I didn't have to drink, and had no physical or mental cravings for alcohol at all. Within a week I had lunch with my family in a pub, and found it quite bizarre to prefer a soft drink (honestly). The following evening I bought some wine for my wife and was happy to pour her a glass or two, without it even crossing my mind that I might want any. Over the weeks that followed my mindset remained the same, and I didn't feel that I was missing out at all.

Despite this amazing change of heart, as the months passed I did find myself drinking again. I was initially very disappointed, depressed almost, feeling that I had failed yet again, totally crashed and burned, and was beyond any further help. But as time passed, I began to realise that this wasn't in fact the abject failure that I had thought. After all, I had learnt the truth about alcohol - the blatant lies of the multi-million pound industry behind it, and the plain fact of alcohol as a foul-tasting poison. This knowledge stayed with me, and was to have a long standing effect on my habits and behaviours. Many months later and I still have no misconceptions whatsoever about alcohol. When I do drink, it is always knowing that I am using a drug, and a dangerous one at that.

Of course there are the obvious questions - is this simply playing with fire? Am I deceiving myself? Is this just another point on the slippery slope of addiction? Only time will tell for sure, but life is certainly very different now. It is hard to believe that I once saw nothing wrong in drinking six or even eight beers every single night of the week.

I am no longer a slave to alcohol, and now life is full of joy and hope that simply did not exist a few months ago. And I am enjoying every single day of it.

I know that I am really just beginning to scratch the surface of these apparently simple changes of perspective, but I can feel the amazing power within. The life potential in this defies conventional logic or reason - everything is possible, and nothing at all is beyond my grasp. Or yours.

Although I couldn't see it at the time, what had happened was this - as my 'higher' self had been growing and expanding, my 'lower' self had remained the same. As time went on, and I continued to grow at the higher level, the gap between the two quickly became a huge gulf. The bigger this got to be, the more I felt like a Jekyll and Hyde character - quite unnerving, I can tell you. You think that you've come so far, only to feel like someone has pulled the rug out from under your feet. You start to question why it is that you are getting in tune with the energies of the universe, but still can't stop yourself from screaming at the kids when you're tired? You are finding your actions becoming increasingly intuitive, resulting in less tension and more success in your life, but still need to drink in order to get through? It doesn't make sense, it feels like you are trying hard, having some success, but then falling by the wayside again. As if you are not good enough to sustain your good work, as if you have tried to develop, but have then hit your ceiling. I simply felt that I had failed, and it was all about to come crashing down around me - I thought I was losing the plot to be honest. The gulf between your higher and lower selves can have a devastating impact on your life, so it is absolutely vital that you see this for what it is.

If you should find yourself in this place, don't panic - you are not going mad, nor have you wasted your time and efforts on the journey so far. It is simply that this gulf is not sustainable. You have reached a point where in order to grow, actually in order to even maintain your higher self at it's current level, you must go back and deal with some of the base stuff - and in doing so, raise your lower self. If you don't, then this gulf can itself become one of the main causes of frustration in your life. And when you are frustrated and dissatisfied, you are more likely to add to your negative behaviour - shout at the kids, squabble with your partner, kick the cat etc. In turn this magnifies the original frustration of your inability to be both Jekyll and Hyde, to live as both increasingly enlightened being, and angry, intolerant man!

It is now apparent that this is a vicious circle which you must break out of, and quickly before you start to self-destruct. So the next step is to look at these base issues, and do something about them. No rocket science here, no bewildering frustration about things not matching up, and no more Jekyll and Hyde. It's just the next step, that's all, just the next stage to be overcome. The fact of knowing this released a lot of my own frustrations, and as a result, let me continue along my path.

So what does come next? What should you do now? Much as I would love to give you the answer to 'life, the universe and everything' in a single sentence, I can't. My truth may not be so different from yours, but the route I take to find it will be. Plenty of people out there are prepared to show you their 'path', but don't mistake it as being yours. However tempting it is, the fact will always remain that you must find your own way.

What I can tell you, is that in order to find your own path, you don't need to believe in anything in particular, you don't have to hold unwavering faith in anyone, and you don't have to be perfect or without fault. You don't have to put your future in the hands of some god or deity, nor do you have to attend any shared place of worship. Actually, you don't have to commit to any specific life changes at all, as the right ones will come to you in their own time. What you do have to accept is that the responsibility for this life is yours, and yours alone. You have to be truly honest with yourself, and to consider what has been written here about truth and perception, the false assumptions we make about our limitations, and how much freedom and power we really have.

And then go. Spread your wings. Create your life.

LEARNING TO FLY

Paul Johnson

17. What Does Success Look Like?

Question - what exactly does success look like? We've all heard of it, most of us have experienced a little of it, and we would all like more of it. But do we really know what it is?

We all have different ideas of what might be required in order to consider ourselves a success. It could be work orientated - climbing the career ladder, getting the nod from senior management or just bringing in some extra money. It could be having a good home - whether large and spacious, or clean, well decorated and homely. It might be family driven - your idea of success might centre around being a good parent, a good aunt or uncle, or being a good role model to younger members of the family.

For the majority, success has always seemed beyond us, somehow out of reach. The idea of this impassable gap between dreams and reality is usually sown in childhood, often by loving parents whose own experiences have taught them not to expect too much from life. Some have also grown up with the additional burden of feeling that whatever they achieve is not good enough, continually trying harder and harder but always feeling inadequate, no matter what their achievements. Again this is something that we tend to grow up with, a matter of absorbing the opinions and views of others as we grow through our most formative years.

One thing that is essential if we are to overcome that which is holding us back, is for us to be bold. Bold enough to look beyond our current horizons. Bold enough to dare to believe that we deserve better. And bold enough to try.

In the film 'Big Fish', the central character has a strange experience - whilst still a child, he is able to see the circumstances of his own death, many years ahead in the future. He goes on to lead a life where he is not afraid to do things because he knows for certain that it is not his time to die. He has seen his own death, but rather than making him afraid, it has actually set him free. As well as facing what appeared to be certain death at times, he also went on to lead a full and interesting life. Not just in terms of achievements - even when this guy didn't know what he wanted to do or be, he would go and look. He would intentionally go and see what was out there, and investigate what experiences life had to offer. I saw this film, and just thought - WOW! Alright, perhaps we need to put the movie stuff to one side - the fearless plunge into dangerous situations would in reality often see you injured or killed. But what of the rest? To be bold enough to satisfy your curiosity, and see what is really out there? To follow your heart without fear, to stay when it's right for you to stay, and leave when it is right for you to leave? And all simply because you know that this is the right thing to do, and aren't afraid to do it? The main character in the film is able to do all of this because he has seen his own death, because he knows that each situation he comes across, however daunting, is not 'his time'.

Aside from being a strangely engaging film, this really made me think. Most of the situations this guy found himself in were not actually life threatening. In the main he just made strong decisions, and did so without any real hesitation, because he wasn't afraid of the unknown. In actual fact, he didn't need to have seen his own death in order to live this way. Think of a life without imagined fears, of making strong decisions and being bold enough to really live? The length of your life, or the nature of your death are not really relevant to this at all, any one of us could live in this way. Ask yourself, as I did - how many chances have I missed through being faint-hearted? How many opportunities have sailed by over the years, simply because I might not have had the nerve to act at the right time? To live with a bold attitude and a good heart is for the better, irrespective of how long you might expect to live. There are important lessons here for each and every one of us. If you haven't seen this exceptional film, I would certainly recommend it.

There is however, a slight drawback with using examples from the movies, as the lead characters are often depicted as being without fear. Perhaps because this is how we imagine that we really ought to be. My experiences in recent years have taught me otherwise - that fear is a part of real life, and should simply be accepted as normal. Fears that are rational, fears that are not, the fears that haunt you for years, or those that just pop up from nowhere and stop you in your tracks - all of these are common, just a natural part of life. There are numerous techniques and strategies that can help free you from the chains that often accompany these feelings, and if you want to learn more about this, I would strongly recommend reading *The Beginners Guide To Darkness* by Geoff Thompson.

The bottom line, however, is that to be without fear is unnatural. Fear is not something to be avoided, rather it is something to be understood, and accepted.

An important point here is that you should not confuse fear with cowardice. I guess we have all heard accounts of courageous people throughout history - it always seemed to me that these men and women were utterly fearless. It is hard to say whether this was because of the way these heroic tales were written, or because of my own feelings of inadequacy. Either way, I always felt so unworthy alongside such heroes, as if I were an inferior specimen - one that should be able to do better, but couldn't. I felt that I had a streak of cowardice running through me, a streak of yellow going right through like Blackpool rock, because I would so often feel scared of situations. Sometimes irrationally, sometimes not, but never entirely sure why. Over time this feeling of cowardice became my 'norm', something I just accepted (incorrectly) as being an unchangeable part of who and what I was.

It is only as I have gotten older that I have begun to understand what courage really is. Forget about the allegedly fearless heroes of days gone by, these are false images, and not what it is about at all. Real courage is simply this - to know what you should do, to be frightened, and then to go on and do it anyway. This is real courage, and don't let anyone ever tell you otherwise. When you find yourself in this position, and you do 'go for it', I can tell you that you don't feel courageous at the time, you feel shit-scared. Just like those supposed fearless heroes from bygone years did, your knees are knocking, you feel sick and rooted to the spot, and the last thing you want to do is to step forwards. It's the same for all of us, just that most won't be honest about it, because it's not thought to be acceptable.

But when you have stepped up, you always know that you did a good thing. Afterwards you feel quietly good about yourself because you did the right thing. You feel a little bit proud of yourself, because this time you didn't wuss-out - instead you saw the moment, felt frightened, and then went on and did it anyway. The funny thing is that afterwards, you don't generally feel **too** proud, because the *doing* part rarely turns out to be all that difficult when you actually take the step. It only ever seems really hard when you're thinking about it, but bottle out at the last minute. Then it becomes mission impossible. But when you do go for it, when you take a deep breath and leap, the reality is never as difficult as you have built it up to be in your mind. In terms of achievements, the fact that you have 'gone for it' should be considered a success in itself, irrespective of the outcome.

Ultimate success however, is not about specific achievements. Instead it is about one thing - **happiness.** Remember, there is no such thing as a perfect world, and there will always be things that we don't like, which have the potential to make us unhappy. The key is to remember that it is our perception of, and our reactions to certain events and experiences that make us unhappy, not the events themselves.

We also frequently go wrong by mistaking material things for happiness, such as money, houses, clothes or cars. Of course we can enjoy those things, but we've all seen enough desperately unhappy rich people in the newspapers to know that money doesn't automatically bring happiness with it. Like most, I'd give it a go, but the reality is that one set of stresses and pressures would simply be replaced by another. So when we can see beyond the superficial, it becomes apparent that happiness is about real fulfilment, genuine contentment. If you can find this, usually accompanied by love for others, then the material things will have less significance for you. As long as you have clothes on your back, and food to go on the table, then these things are of much less importance. When you attain this perspective, you find that the recipe for true happiness is to have love for those around you, and not lose sight of this as we go through our day-to-day lives.

It has been noted by many wise men that have gone before, that true happiness is right there in front of us throughout our entire lives, waiting for us. But we each have to decide when we are ready to reach out and take it.

Choose Life

We all find it difficult to stay firmly on this path to an improved self, and often need some sort of framework to keep us on track. We might use goal-setting to help us to achieve, however when we reach our goals, it is never quite as good as we imagined. The initial high might be great, the rush of excitement exhilarating, but it doesn't last all that long. Following the excitement is a slight lack of satisfaction, or an impatience to get onto the next thing, so we push on for that next step, and the next, and the next. And so it goes on. It is important to take the time to appreciate what you have achieved, but also to recognise and accept that your journey is one without end. So you must always keep moving, keep working, at whatever pace is sustainable for you.

Someone said to me recently that the impermanence of achievements surely makes them irrelevant, that we are perhaps mistaken if we commit so much time and energy to achieving things that in themselves are only temporary, and that the sense of achievement that comes with it also passes. However the point of aiming towards and achieving something is *not* the goal itself, but rather the change that happens to you whilst going through the process. The growth that happens when you push through disappointment and failure, brush aside 'normal' restrictions and start making things happen. There is no question that some achievements will only give satisfaction for a certain length of time, and that others may not even be what you had anticipated. But the internal growth is something that you take with you, and which feeds into your development along the way. Happiness and satisfaction are both things that are ultimately to be found within yourself, rather than through external achievements or acquisitions.

The only real mistake you can make on this journey is to stop. Your mind will inevitably play games and present all kinds of apparently justifiable reasons to slow down your progress, and prevent you from pushing through your boundaries. When this happens, you might find yourself thinking of putting your plans to one side, or saying *I'll start again when the summer's here*, or *when work's not so busy*, or whatever. When a reason like this comes along, you must take a long hard look at it before you allow yourself to stop and lose momentum. There may be times when you genuinely have no choice, but before you stop, make sure that the reason isn't an excuse, isn't just the fear factor in a new disguise. If you have already stopped, then keep the break short and get back to it as soon as possible. Restarting can be difficult when the momentum has gone, so surround yourself with motivation and inspiration. Pick up that book, put on that CD or DVD, or go talk to friends and family if you are lucky enough to have the right sort of people around you. Whatever it takes, get yourself built up with inspiration and enthusiasm, and get started again as soon as possible.

So to go back to the question posed – what exactly is success? As you will have gathered by now, I believe that **success is simply to live a life of happiness.**

And what is happiness? To recap, let's first be clear about what it isn't - happiness has nothing to do with what you have in material terms, about the state of your bank balance or the size of your car. **Happiness is a *state of mind*.** It is about your self image - your perception of who you are. It is also about your relationships with those you love - of how your thoughts and actions flow with life, and also with the lives of those around you.

Our journey takes us onwards and upwards towards this success. We might sometimes feel disorientated, or that we are losing ground and going backwards, but as long as you continue to push forwards and live with a positive mindset, then such negative feelings will soon pass. When living in tune with life, we are always moving forward, although we often have to grasp difficult lessons along the way. Mistakes do happen, and should be expected from time to time, however it is important to remember that we really do learn more from our mistakes than our successes. Strange then, that we view mistakes so negatively. Instead you need to start redefining your mistakes, and look upon them as learning opportunities. Not meant as 'self-help waffle', but by thinking of these events in a different context, even by simply referring to them in your mind by a different (positive) name, will make a huge difference. Incredibly, the negatives associated with mistakes are lost, and the positives start to pour from these opportunities. Again this is a simple change in perspective, but the benefits quickly begin to appear, as if by magic.

Choose Life

Above all else, remember that just getting through those learning opportunities (as many as it might take), is the way to reach the next milestone on this, your journey towards an increasingly happy and successful life.

Paul Johnson

18. Accepting Success

Successful achievements come along in a wide variety of shapes and sizes - different things for different people. I started to find some degree of success with my writing, however this was very difficult to share with others, as I was afraid of their reactions. There I was, secretly bashing away at the keyboard in stolen moments, keeping it hidden. Ashamed almost, as if it were some sort of dirty secret. When I did talk to close family and friends, I got all sorts of different reactions, including a few that I hadn't expected. Some people are thrilled to see you take on something new, but others will be negative and sceptical. There are those who are seem determined to discredit you, and others who are apparently jealous of any success you might be having, as if it were some sort of comment on their own failings.

I knew one guy who was apparently happy for me, but then couldn't wait until I had finished telling my news before he talked all over it with stories of his own plans and achievements. Sad really, as I was no threat to his own success, but he seemed to take it that way. Others would have a joke with me, mocking my 'new found' knowledge, with an edge that was beyond normal banter. I found this bewildering, and very negative. As a result I no longer talk to these people about anything new. It's not all doom and gloom though - some friends that I had expected to say little and pass over it all quite quickly, were in fact really happy for me, and wanted to know all about it. So, it can be quite a mixed bag - you think that you know people, but when you have had even a small success, you may be surprised by some of their reactions. It is a shame that it sometimes comes with the odd disappointment, but perhaps this is when you find out who your real friends are.

A while ago I was talking to a guy who has been a massive inspiration to me, indirectly through his work over many years, and also more recently with some personal advice on my own writing. He had been kind enough to read an article I had written, and then advised me to go and expand it into a book. So, I went away and wrote (and wrote and wrote). The weeks passed, and I went back to him and said *I've expanded it, got fourteen thousand words now - job's a good 'un, right?* The conversation that followed was both positive and encouraging, however he did point out (very gently) that a book would normally be at least three or four times that length. But hey, I've got broad shoulders, much better to get honest advice, I can cope with that. Besides, so much else was positive, this guy thought that I had a future as a writer - heady stuff coming from an established author! So I decided not to worry about it, and spent the rest of the evening quite excited about the possibilities that had appeared before me.

But the following day comes and I'm very low. A future in writing? That would mean more work, more ideas, more books...? Hang on a minute, how am I going to write something else? It's all good and well tinkering around at my own pace, but imagine if someone actually asked me to produce something? *Ok, Mr. Johnson, if you're as good as you say you are, we'd like you to do some work for us. If you could just knock off a quick ten thousand words, we're looking for a short story that is both motivational and inspirational. Perhaps you could let us see the first draft in a month's time?*

Can you imagine?

Oh my god, oh my god, oh my god...I'm panicking... what the hell am I going to do? It's all good and well standing up and claiming to be a credible writer, but I feel like I've already bitten off more than I can possibly chew. I haven't finished my first book yet, and I'm in blind panic about my next project. I don't even know what it's going to be yet, come to think of it I'm really not sure I should have started all of this. Don't think I can keep up with this, it's too big for me - I can't even deliver against yesterday's rush of enthusiasm, oh my god, what on earth was I thinking??

Arrgghhh!!

At this point I had written a total of about fourteen thousand words, across twelve short chapters. A day or two earlier, I had told myself that if a prospective publisher were to tell me that my work was good, but needed to grow to twenty thousand words, then I would say *sorry, but no - this thing has already grown to it's natural size, can't be done. Not possible, it just hasn't got any more in it.* Thankfully (in the end), the advice I was given wasn't that I needed a few more pages, in fact it seemed I needed at least three times as much as I had currently done, if not more. Talk about being knocked for six... I did genuinely appreciate the honest advice (no point in any other sort), but even so I just couldn't get my head around this. Mentally, I spent the next day on the floor, moaning to myself that I just couldn't do it. At least forty thousand words, a massive amount of work. At one point I'm sure he mentioned fifty to sixty thousand!

Breathe, just breathe...

It wasn't just the volume that bothered me, it was also the quality. I was not convinced that it was viable to treble the page count whilst maintaining the quality, and it became very clear that any future publishing deal was a long, long way off. There was so much to do, such a mountain to climb if I was ever to complete my first book. And I was doing what? Panicking because I didn't have any ideas for my *second* book? Stupid...

The fear was unreal. I felt like throwing the towel in, partly because I couldn't conceive of my work growing to this size, but also because someone else had said there was a future to this, that I could and would produce more good quality work. They weren't asking for proof either, this was an opinion based on what they had already seen. That being the case, then why was it that I needed proof of my ability to produce future work? Simple - because I couldn't believe in myself as a writer, not really, not in my heart of hearts. I felt like packing it all in, and was almost defeated by the beginnings of some small success.

Finally the resilience kicks in - time to shift my thinking here, and harness the positive in all of this. So let's have a look, let's have a think about what I've got here, how I've structured my work. I realise that I'm still approaching this as a very long article... time to move things on, to see this as the outline of a 'proper' book for the first time. Out comes pen and paper, and I let my imagination run free, let myself dare to believe. Half an hour later and the whole thing has a different structure. I have now split the book into five different parts, to have around twenty chapters - the existing ones all need expanding, and the others are not yet written. But guess what? I can see the book. I can actually see the book - it has become viable in my mind. This isn't about suddenly writing a lot more words, I still have the same fourteen thousand. But now instead of being a 'nearly completed something', it has become the outline of a bigger, bolder project - some of it part-written, some of it just the beginnings of ideas, but crucially this was no longer an article. Thanks to some rather timely advice, a mini-project that was running out of steam suddenly became transformed into a genuinely viable book, and with this I was filled from the top of my head to my toes with energy, enthusiasm and inspiration.

It was at this point that I came up against a very important question - if you don't truly believe in yourself, why should anyone else?

Although I was now enthusiastically writing on a regular basis, and had the beginnings of a book set out in a workable framework, I still saw myself as a beginner - you know, giving it a go, but saying to myself - *I'm just having a little play with this, maybe something will come of it, maybe it won't. No great problem if it doesn't work out, 'cos I'm just having a little dabble.*

I kept telling myself this, and also kept telling other people the same thing. That way I wasn't setting expectations (theirs or mine), and therefore couldn't really fail, couldn't be disappointed if it didn't work out. You know the way these negative thoughts work - *none of us like rejection, reach too far and you run the risk of crashing down in abject failure.* I think this was more pronounced because I couldn't see myself as a writer at all - in my head this was extremely pretentious. Although I really wanted to write, and to be a writer, I just couldn't get my head around it.

Slowly I began to see that as long as I kept telling myself that I was just dabbling, then dabbling was all that I would ever do. The time had come - if I was ever to become a 'proper' writer, then I was going to have to take a deep breath and start thinking of myself as one. Can I or can't I? Am I or am I not? This was a big choice, and would prove to be another self-fulfilling prophecy.

It was a huge leap from where my head was at the time, so to make it do-able I broke it down into much smaller pieces. Never mind being a full-time writer, raking in millions or anything too far-fetched - I decided to stick with the fundamentals, i.e. that I couldn't see myself as a writer at all, that it was all pretentious bollocks etc. Then at last the penny finally dropped - hang on a minute, if I am sitting down and bashing at the keyboard a few times a week, then I already AM a writer by definition.

It didn't matter at this point what I was producing, how many words or even what the quality was - as I said, this wasn't about seeing myself as a successful, published writer, it was about being able to get my head around being a writer at all. So at the point of realisation, I had by definition already been a writer for several months. Even the fact I felt uncomfortable about that couldn't change it - I was writing on a regular basis, therefore I was a writer. WOW. I still am writing on a regular basis, and it still amazes me to think that I AM a writer. What a fantastic feeling - but at least now I can accept this, and enjoy the rush that comes with it.

Don't try to bypass this first stage of acceptance, because if you can't see yourself as being a writer, a teacher, a mountain climber or whatever it is that you want to be, then you won't ever become one.

The moment I stood up and said I AM A WRITER, it felt like I was challenging the whole world, daring them to try and flatten me, to bring me back down to earth. But without that self-belief and commitment, there is no way that your dream will ever come to fruition. As it was, the only thing my previous mindset had given me was a ready made excuse in case it all went wrong - *hey, I never said I was that bothered if nothing came of this.* But aside from saving a bit of face, exactly what good would that do me? I would still have failed miserably. Bottling out because of the fear of failure is bad enough, but because you are frightened of succeeding...?

So, scary or otherwise, I realised that I had to change my thinking. I was going to have to believe in myself, if I ever expected anyone else to. And now I do. I don't claim to be infallible on this score - I think the ups and downs are just part of human nature, so for the time being I will continue to carry a spare pair of pants with me. But it has become do-able, success now seems like a reasonable outcome, and sometimes even a quite likely one.

This whole process is quite incredible. Most of the limitations that hold us back are self-created, much like the ones that almost made me throw the towel in a while back. These self-imposed parameters actually govern what you can conceive as being within your power - what you have accepted as your limitations will determine your reality, and then define what seems to be possible/impossible. Where these boundaries have been in place for many years, it can be difficult to shift your thinking, even more so if they are boundaries that you grew up with. But even so, they are only thoughts, and are therefore not real unless you acknowledge them as being real. And even if you have, they can be changed with a little effort. So you can think this through, find out what it is that you think is holding you back, which hurdles are 'impossible' to overcome, and then think it through again, only this time with a different mindset. You will find an answer, and it will probably lie in examining some of the things that you have either set or accepted as 'sensible' limits. Once you change these boundaries, your thinking expands, and then your whole perspective changes with it.

As your perspective expands, the key is then to recognise and embrace this change, and accept it as being part of the 'new you'. This is not a brand new you, not some unrecognisable alter-ego that you have just invented and given radically different values and beliefs. Too much too quickly, and the 'old you' will usually reject this 'new you', the result being a demoralising reversion to type - a rapid retreat back to former thinking, habits and behaviours. Instead think of this as a process of refining that which already exists. Then at each stage of development you will be able to recognise and accept the new model as simply being a new and improved version of yourself.

Although this may sound deceptively simple, it is mind-blowing to experience. It is almost spiritual in nature, and it is true to say that nothing will ever feel the same again, and nothing will ever seem impossible again. It's straightforward enough, but also life-changing. The scale of the potential within this is so awesome, that it has to be felt rather than described. It is absolutely amazing, but please don't just take my word for it - get out there and try this for yourself.

Choose Life

If we are to continue to grow, then it is important that we do accept and embrace our achievements at each milestone along the way. Sometimes this feels as if it should be forbidden, as if it is being 'big-headed', but remember you are only ever comparing yourself against yourself, which is never wrong. The only person that can now cause you to fail is you, and the way through this is to challenge the negative side of your self image. Allow yourself to believe that you can succeed, that you are worthy of success, in fact that you **deserve** to succeed in your goals. At this stage there is no need to worry about success feeding the ego excessively, as we have grown way beyond this.

So give yourself permission to succeed, become comfortable with the idea of being a success, and then make sure you settle for nothing less.

19. Choose Life

Some years ago I saw a documentary about the war in Vietnam, and how certain drugs were given to some of the American soldiers. The intention was that they should lose their natural reluctance to take life, hence turning the soldiers into more effective killing machines. To explain the effects of one drug in particular, the narrator described how we each have unique 'filters' within our minds, through which we define that which we understand and accept as reality. These filters help us to sort through and dismiss much of the information that is coming in through our senses, and make some sort of coherent sense of what remains. We do this by making a comparison between the incoming information and our stored knowledge and accepted version of reality, which in turn enables us to make decisions. It was said that without these filters, we would be unable to cope with the massive volume of information that we are constantly picking up from our environment.

For example, take a walk down the street in which you live. Most of the information coming into your brain will relate to what you can see and hear, with other senses usually playing a lesser role. The sheer quantity of available data is staggering. Imagine **really** looking, seeing the wealth of visual details from everything around you - the individual bricks that make up each house in the street, the different cars parked on the road, the contrasting styles and individual content of each garden, the wind moving the trees at the end of the road, and how each leaf moves differently from the others, but in rhythm with it's neighbours. And so on. If we were to take all of this in, it really would be overwhelming. So instead, the brain will usually ignore most of the information, and our attention will only be drawn to things that are substantially different from what we already know. At other times we are so preoccupied with our thoughts that we walk or drive as if in a daze, and notice nothing of our surroundings.

In the TV documentary, it was said that the effects of the drug given to the American soldiers was not to change these filters, but to remove them completely.

Can you imagine losing your accepted understanding of reality?

Can you imagine taking in absolutely everything, all at once??

These filters generally work in our favour, however they can also work against us. Our inability to see what is right in front of our nose is a major problem, and impacts on lives and relationships across the world. Take, for example, a couple that have been married for many years, and imagine a situation that you might hear on the evening news - suppose they were in their local supermarket and the woman disappeared without trace. Nowhere to be seen, no obvious reason, and no hints or clues to go on. By the time the police arrived, what are the chances of her husband being able to describe what clothes she had on? If she was wearing her glasses or not? If her hair was up or down? Our tendency to take familiar things for granted is a dangerous factor in any relationship.

This is an important point, as enlightenment is about seeing what we really have in this world, and understanding the immeasurable value within. Happiness is to be found in those things that are already there, all around you, such as your partner or children, your parents and friends, or your pets at home. The trees in the park, the grass blowing in the wind, and the shapes of the clouds in the sky. The things that are so close that we no longer look, or see what wondrous lives we have. We need to dust off the familiar and the apparently mundane, and see what incredible jewels lie just beneath the surface. Not only as an occasional fleeting glimpse within the hectic rush of modern living, but to be able to feel this, and value it on a daily basis. To me, this is the real meaning of enlightenment. Ultimate success is to have clear sight of these most valuable of treasures which have been in front of our noses throughout the entire journey - hidden away in plain view the whole time.

Now we have reached the point on our journey where this realisation has hit us between the eyes. We have reached enlightenment through the mundane, and feel that life can never be the same again. Granted, we realise that old habits die hard, and know that we will need to work to maintain this new perspective, but still, we know that a milestone has been reached, that this has been a major turning point in our lives. To have reached this point is amazing. But what comes next?

When I was signed off with stress, this was the longest period of time I had taken off work since leaving school all those years ago. And it was difficult to go back. For the first time I had caught a glimpse of another life, another possible future - one that didn't include the nine to five office routine that I had always assumed would be mine until old and grey. I would walk down the street and see the trees, hear the birds. I would see beauty in the reflections of car headlights on the wet road, and sense the wonder of life in everything and everyone. I felt compassion for those around me when they were in the wrong, instead of getting annoyed with them. After all, they weren't in the same place as me - I was fortunate to have this clarity of vision, and see things for what they really were. I could empathise with people who were upset or angry about a given situation, and understand their feelings. However I could also see a much wider perspective, and how they were being held back by their emotional responses and reactive approach to life. A feeling of understanding and real compassion, as wide as the Universe itself.

So I went back to work, only to find that my new perspective felt quite strange. I felt somehow out of place. It was really trippy - not unpleasant, but odd, like I had somehow slipped into an alternative reality. I would sometimes sense people looking at me as if I had said something peculiar, thinking I was making some sort of odd joke that they didn't really get, when in fact I had just found myself with a rather different view of things. They might have thought I was out there on another planet, but it all made perfect sense to me.

After a while I began to wonder about this new perspective that I had taken to be some degree of enlightenment, as it didn't seem to line up with certain aspects of my life, particularly at work. It became apparent that the situation might not be sustainable. However, I then found myself gently coming back down to something resembling normal life. I did worry that I might lose the insights that had been earned through my experience and pain, but as usual, this was a worry about nothing. I'm not out there on another planet any more, but having returned to Earth, I find that I am still seeing things a little differently - not spaced out or trippy, but still content in the knowledge that nothing will ever be quite the same again. I am looking through a different set of filters now, ones that let me see more clearly, and with a wider perspective. I'm sure this process will happen over and over, with my vision clearing more each time, however I am grateful that these filters didn't come off in one go, as I am quite sure my sanity would have disappeared with them. It didn't do the guys in Vietnam much good, if I remember rightly…

So that's the whole journey - from the mundane to the spiritual, and then back again to the mundane. It has been described in this way by many wise men over the ages, but it means something wholly different when you have been there yourself. When you return to your familiar day-to-day life, things look somehow different, with so much of exceptional value in your life that it seems difficult to understand how you couldn't see it before. What might not be so immediately obvious, is the knock-on effect - you may think this only affects yourself, but like the proverbial ripple in the pond, there is a direct impact on those around you. You will start (without trying) to share this perspective, this natural balance and vision. Although it is certainly true that not everyone is ready to listen, you are able to lead by example, and take a subtle approach by simply being yourself, and living in tune with your increasingly positive values and perspective. This has an unmistakeable affect on others, especially those close to you. And serving others in this way is ultimately what this journey is about.

The thing to remember now is how important it is not to take your eye off the ball. It's all too easy to slip and fall back into old habits, especially when they have been a way of life for some time. So make sure you keep your awareness up and spot the warnings signs - they should be as familiar as an old friend by now! And when you do see or feel your own warning signs, then take action, and do so promptly and firmly. After all, you haven't been through all of this for nothing, have you?

But what should you do when the pace of modern living threatens to disrupt your new-found state of mind? Just open your eyes - literally. You can use this most powerful of senses to bring yourself fully into the present. Focus your eyes and attention on whatever is around you, and search out the detail - whether it is in the leaves on a tree, patterns in your wallpaper, or the grain lines in a wooden table. By bringing yourself firmly into the present in this way, you disengage from the thoughts which were creating stress, or from the discomfort of trying to go faster than the speed of life. You instead find yourself re-tuning back into the proper flow of things. In your most natural of states. And after a while this becomes a pleasure in itself.

At this point it is important to reflect and remember just how far you have come. When stress is running your life, you can easily feel like a dead man walking, like you've lost sight of what it's all about. In fact it's about quality of life - years clocked up mean nothing if you have no depth of joy, if you don't enjoy something of each day. But you can change this, you can do something different. This life is of your own making, or at least it can be. To choose your own path now, away from the expectations of friends, family, workmates or whoever, and go where you choose, is very liberating. A little scary perhaps, but also very exciting. To realise you can finally walk your own path, and that it doesn't at all mean leaving people behind. To realise that your perceived fears and restrictions are either of your own making, or they come from the blinkered expectations of others. And to realise that these thoughts can be discarded if you wish, and need only apply if you want them to.

WOW.

Remember - the fact is that we often can't change the world around us, but we can change how we interact with it. Know that our stress is ultimately caused within, by how we react to things that happen in the world around us, and because we have the power to change ourselves, we can therefore get to the root of the problem. We are all responsible for our own experience of life, and our own quality of existence. And when you pick this up, when you accept this responsibility, then not only will your own life change, but you will also have a profound effect on those around you.

Simplicity is a theme that has run throughout these pages. It seems that most of the unnecessary complications are created by ourselves, and a better life has little to do with building anything new, but is instead about stripping away the unnecessary. Finding that which is already inside.

The starting point however is one that we haven't yet identified, although it is no more than a simple choice. A choice to be made just before the point of accepting responsibility, and one which is often overlooked. This is the point at which we stop worrying about the detail of where we are, where we need to go, or how we will get there. This is the point that we make the decision to **choose life** - a better life in every way from this day forward. This brings with it an implicit commitment to follow a positive route from this point, to consciously steer clear of the negatives in this world. If we leap past this in our haste to make good, then the positive actions we try to employ will often flounder, as we need a firm mental resolve to be the solid foundation on which we build the rest of our lives.

If you aren't happy with your life, if you are fighting yourself day after day, or struggling to break away from ingrained habits or behaviours, then this choice is your starting point. If you recognise parts of yourself within these pages, then again, this choice is the starting point for a better life and a more fulfilling future.

So go on, make the commitment in your decision right now, open up all of the possibilities and the incredible potential that lies dormant within each and every one of us.

Choose Life.

www.ingramcontent.com/pod-product-compliance
Lightning Source LLC
Chambersburg PA
CBHW031201270326
41931CB00006B/364